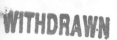

Behavioral Habilitation through Proactive Programming

Behavioral Habilitation through Proactive Programming

by

Gail S. Bernstein, Ph.D.,
Jon P. Ziarnik, Ph.D.,
Eric H. Rudrud, Ph.D.,
John F. Kennedy Child Development Center
University of Colorado Health Sciences Center

and
Laura A. Czajkowski, M.S.
Department of Psychology
Utah State University

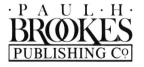
·P A U L·H·
BROOKES
PUBLISHING CO

Baltimore • London

Paul H. Brookes Publishing Co.
Post Office Box 10624
Baltimore, Maryland 21204

Typeset by The Composing Room of Michigan, Inc. (Grand Rapids)
Manufactured in the United States of America by
Universal Lithographers, Inc. (Cockeysville, Maryland)

Library of Congress Cataloging in Publication Data
Main entry under title:

Behavioral habilitation through proactive
    programming.

    Bibliography: p.
    Includes index.
    1. Developmentally disabled—Rehabilitation.
2. Social work education.   3. Paraprofessionals
in social service—Training of.   I. Bernstein,
Gail S., 1947–   . [DNLM: 1. Behavior
therapy.   2. Education, Special.   3. Handicapped.   4. Rehabilitation. LC 4015 B419]
HV3004.B44   362.3'83   81-10134
ISBN 0-933716-19-2   AACR2

Contents

Introduction

The last decade has brought startling advances in knowledge, philosophy, and, most importantly, training techniques for developmentally disabled individuals. We have moved from the human warehouses of recent memory to the broad-based habilitation programs of today. However, our capacity to educate direct care service providers regarding new training techniques and new knowledge is still limited. Colleges and universities, firmly rooted in a liberal arts tradition, are slow to react to new person-power needs. As a result, many direct care staff in the field have had no formal education in providing services to developmentally disabled clients. The problems of service delivery are further compounded by the increasing number of community-based programs dispersed over wide areas. Few of these programs have access to professional resources within university or institutional settings.

Behavioral Habilitation through Proactive Programming has been written to help direct care staff and other service providers who lack a specific background in training the developmentally disabled. The contents of the book are an outgrowth of a curriculum for staff employed in community programs that was developed by the authors while working in a staff development program at the University of South Dakota. Thus, the material is practical and can be directly applied by the reader. Also, each chapter includes learning objectives, reference materials, and exercises to help the reader master the contents.

Proactive Programming is based on a holistic model that stresses that techniques of behavior change are of limited value unless the practitioner is equally skilled in behavioral assessment, prioritizing and selecting habilitation goals, and identifying appropriate training content. Habilitation training is conceived of as a process of moving the client from one place to another along a continuum, similar to a trip or journey. This book is divided into seven organizational units that ask the basic programmatic questions: "Why are we going?" "Where are we going?" "Where are we presently?" and "How do we get there?"

Unit I, Foundations, asks the question: "Why are we going?" The habilitation journey begins here with an explanation of the proactive philosophy and a discussion of important legal and historical events that influence current services. These theoretical underpinnings form the foundations of modern service delivery.

The second unit (Individualized Program Planning: Where Are We Going?) stresses the importance of clear goal setting and involvement of the habilitation team in achieving goals. One major problem of human services programs is that they attempt to meet too many broad social goals simultaneously. Often the end result is that none of the goals are met. Unless there is a clear sense of "where we are going" the probability of reaching goals is greatly reduced.

Just knowing where we are going is not enough. Before any journey can begin, we must also know "Where are we?" Unit III, Behavioral Assessment, stresses the importance of accurate assessment of pretraining behaviors and continuous monitoring of training progress in order to demonstrate program effectiveness.

Unit IV (Behavior Management: How Do We Get There?) is unique among publications of this type. In addition to stressing concepts (e.g., what is a reinforcer?) and the application of specific techniques (e.g., how to reinforce), the reader is taught a system of analyzing behaviors and evaluating programmatic options. We firmly believe that learning only specific techniques is of limited value. For example, learning how to use timeout to reduce a client's tantrums does not teach the reader how to determine program effectiveness, how to modify existing programs, how to deal with another client's tantrums, or that the use of timeout is just one component of a total habilitation program. Thus, this unit emphasizes strategies for analyzing behaviors and presents models to aid in decision-making.

Successful habilitation also involves utilizing curriculum materials to aid in teaching new skills to clients. Service providers are literally deluged with materials. Unit V (Instructional Materials: Helping Us Get There) is designed to assist the reader in evaluating the appropriateness and potential effectiveness of available materials. Additionally, guidelines for the adaptation of instructional materials are provided.

The first five units provide direct care staff with the basics of services to clients. However, the provision of quality services involves more than well-trained staff. To enhance the likelihood of success of the habilitation journey, the organization that employs the staff must also be supportive. It is our contention that, when other things are equal, the basic reason for the differences in the quality of care between programs is attributable to the administrative climate of the organization. Unit VI (The Proactive Organization: Support for Going) extends our knowledge of learning and motivation to administrative activities.

The last unit (Resource Utilization: Traveler's Aid) is designed to inform the reader about community resources, the potential involvement of other professionals as program allies, and sources of useful information.

Clients, staff, administrators, and organizations embark on the journey of service delivery. We hope that our philosophy will provide a road map leading to successful client programming. Detours can and will be eliminated with a solid and proactive approach. Additionally, we hope that our road map makes the habilitation journey less stressful and less time consuming.

Acknowledgments

Much of the content and organization for this book, as well as the philosophy on which it is based, was conceived and implemented while the authors were employed as the members of the Division of Training, Center for the Developmentally Disabled (UAP), at the University of South Dakota. During our time there, South Dakota increased emphasis on community-based services. One major function of the Division of Training was to provide technical assistance and staff training for these programs.

Staff training in a largely rural, northern state requires considerable travel over vast distances in uncertain weather. Over a four-year period, nearly 20% of the authors' time was spent in cars or planes simply getting to community programs. Despite the blizzards, mechanical breakdowns, grounded planes, and nights in motels, we each appreciate the enthusiasm and humor that each of us has been able to maintain. For the past several years it has been our rare good fortune to work as colleagues who truly function as a team. We come from very different backgrounds. The melding of our ideas into a common theme was the result of years of continuous give and take among ourselves. If this book serves its purpose, it will be largely because four very opinionated people were willing to listen to and learn from each other, to praise where appropriate, and to provide constructive criticism when necessary. We are therefore pleased to acknowledge that this book was totally collaborative. The order of the authors was randomly chosen and is not reflective of differential contributions.

We are particularly indebted to Thomas Scheinost, Program Administrator for the South Dakota Office of Developmental Disabilities. He is truly an exceptional administrator. Without his continued belief in and support of the Division of Training, this book simply would not have been possible. Additionally, the Office of Developmental Disabilities field staff—Tim Kosier, Don Wetrich, Pat Wilson, and Patti Miles—consistently facilitated our efforts to improve staff competence. We also extend our thanks to the South Dakota Association of Adjustment Services for their involvement. Finally, we would like to thank all the direct care staff who participated in our training programs, provided helpful feedback, and encouraged our efforts.

Three other people made contributions to this book and our training effort. Jake Mauldin was an integral part of our team for an all too brief period. He nevertheless made substantial contributions to the development of our program, by providing a moral grounding for much of our work. Janie Rudrud was largely responsible for the development of our resource library, was involved in many phases of our media productions, and helped immensely in searching out needed reference information. Thony Jones, who was also a part of our team for a short time, brought new perspectives to our work that are reflected in this text.

We are indebted to the many professionals who have influenced our collective and individual thinking during each of our careers. Some of them deserve special mention here. Dr. Bernstein would like to thank Dr. William I. Gardner of the University of

Wisconsin–Madison, whose conceptual approach to human problems has had a major impact on the development of our system, and Dr. Orv C. Karan, also of the University of Wisconsin–Madison, for his thoughtful support. Dr. Ziarnik would like to thank Dr. Robert Weiss of the University of Oregon, who started his interest in behavioral psychology, and Dr. James Mikawa of the University of Nevada-Reno and Dr. Michael O'Leary of the University of Washington for providing a community-oriented structure for his interest. He is also indebted to Dr. Lee Koeningsberg and Howard Rosen of the Federal Regional Office of Developmental Disabilities, who were so readily helpful to a young, naive administrator.

Dr. Ziarnik came to the University of Colorado Health Sciences Center less than a year before this manuscript was completed, and Drs. Bernstein and Rudrud arrived only two months before our deadline. We owe special thanks to Dr. William Frankenburg, the Director of the John F. Kennedy Child Development Center, for his encouragement for this project and, particularly, for his patience while new staff devoted large blocks of time to completing this text.

Finally, we have been particularly blessed by the availability of extremely competent and good-natured typists. Only other authors can fully appreciate how much we owe to Patti Thedens, who typed most of the manuscript from unbelievably rough copy. We are also indebted to Jolene Constance and Diane Wusteman for their assistance with the typing.

About the Authors

Gail S. Bernstein received her B.S. (1968), M.S. (1975), and Ph.D. (1978) from the University of Wisconsin-Madison. Prior to beginning her graduate studies she taught high school and worked in both a group home for disturbed adolescents and an institution for mentally retarded adults. During most of her graduate work she was a case coordinator for a program designed to develop habilitation procedures for severely developmentally disabled individuals. She is currently with the Division of Community Education and Technical Assistance at the John F. Kennedy Child Development Center and is Assistant Professor, Department of Preventive Medicine, both at the University of Colorado Health Sciences Center. Her interests and activities include provision of staff training and case consultation, research in staff training, behavioral assessment, and organizational development.

Jon P. Ziarnik received his B.S. (1972) from the University of Oregon, and Ph.D. (1976) from the University of Nevade-Reno. His doctorate is in clinical psychology with an emphasis in adult psychopathology. His present interests are in administration and organizational development. In 1976 he went to South Dakota to begin the Division of Training, a state-wide staff training and technical assistance project, where he served as Director until 1980. Presently, he is Associate Director of the Division of Community Education and Technical Assistance at the John F. Kennedy Child Development Center and Assistant Professor, Department of Preventive Medicine, at the University of Colorado Health Sciences Center.

Eric H. Rudrud received his B.S. (1972) from Colorado State University, and M.S. (1974) and Ph.D. (1978) from Utah State University. He has had experience working with developmentally disabled individuals of all ages in a variety of clinical settings, including public school systems, state institutions, university affiliated programs, and private nonprofit agencies. His areas of interest include applied behavior analysis, organizational development, child development, and biofeedback. He is currently with the Division of Community Education and Technical Assistance at the John F. Kennedy Child Development Center and is Assistant Professor, Department of Preventive Medicine, both at the University of Colorado Health Sciences Center. His activities include provision of staff training and case consultation and development of training materials.

Laura A. Czajkowski received her B.A. (1972) from Hunter College and M.S. (1973) from Indiana State University. Her interests include applied behavior analysis, behavioral medicine, staff training, and curriculum development. She has had experience working with handicapped individuals in public schools, institutions, community-based programs, and hospitals. Until 1980 she was project director of a BEH Inservice Training Grant at the Center for the Developmentally Disabled, Division of Training, University of South Dakota. She is currently at Utah State University where she is enrolled in the doctoral program in psychology and employed at the Exceptional Child Center.

Unit I

Foundations
Why Are We Going?

Chapter 1

The Proactive Approach

OBJECTIVES

To be able to:
1. Define the difference between proactive and reactive programming.
2. List the six characteristics of a proactive staff person.
3. Take reactively stated client programs and redefine them in proactive terms.
4. Identify reactive aspects of your own training techniques and alter them so that they are proactive.

There is a common problem found throughout human service organizations and programs. That is, the system of services that has developed is largely reactive. It is structured to respond to events after these events have begun or occurred. This is true for many people-oriented programs, such as health care services (with extensive hospital and emergency services but less emphasis placed on how to get and stay healthy), and insurance programs (with disability benefits but little payoff for people who remain productive workers). In developmental disabilities we see system-wide reactive priorities, with efforts in training and education of clients but few coordinated programs to reduce the incidence of developmental disabilities. A reactive approach is not entirely negative in that it does meet many of the "felt needs" of people. Simply put, "felt needs" are those problems that people rarely think about until they happen. However, when they do happen, people want immediate solutions, as in the case of illness or natural disaster. On the other hand, a reactive system has certain built-in disadvantages. Any entirely reactive system is very costly, inefficient, and self-perpetuating because it does not directly solve the causes of problems. Using a bucket to catch drips from a leaky roof solves the immediate problem of a wet floor, but does not fix the basic problem of the leak. Reactivity is simply solving problems as they come up.

If we wish to reduce recurring problems, it is time to place emphasis on total human service systems—that is, those that have the capacity to both react to the effects of problems and solve the origin of problems. The need for a total approach is particularly true in developmental disabilities. We have a great deal of knowledge about the origin of problems and about the origins of various handicapping conditions, but we have yet to fully apply our knowledge to the prevention of developmental disabilities (Drash, Boyd, & Stolberg, 1979). We all know of cases where clients collect more money in disability benefit programs than they could make if they were fully employed. Thus, in some cases, a client is reluctant to become rehabilitated to his or her economic disadvantage. The origin of this problem is the structure of our benefit programs (Bernstein & Karan, 1979). We are quick to call for the development of community-based programs but ignore the fact that there are few personnel trained to provide services in community-based programs (Magrab & Elder, 1979). Thus, we have facilities and legislative mandates to provide quality programs, but encounter difficulties finding experienced staff to carry out the programs. Such reactivity is even found in the national history of developmental disabilities, when we entered the age of planning before we developed shared goals (Krishef, 1978). After you are familiar with the goal-planning process (Chapter 4), you will know that the first phase of planning is always the development of goals.

Exercise

1-1. Bill Brown is a 38-year-old resident of a small town in South Dakota. He is mentally retarded, with an IQ score of 65, and has been in vocational and community living training at a community-based day activity program for the last six years. Prior to that time Bill resided at the state institution. Bill's father is deceased and his mother lives in a small town two hours away. Bill has progressed well in his vocational training, but his progress in community living training has been slow, although steady. The community living staff judge that Bill is unable to live independently and is in need of further training. Bill readily agrees; however, Bill's new job pays $424.50 per month (minimum wage) and as a result he is ineligible for a number of programs, including SSDI, Medicaid, and Medicare. Additionally, he is ineligible for Title XX, which previously funded his community living training. As a result, the facility must charge Bill for the needed training ($230 per month plus room and board, another $180 per month). This total of $410, when subtracted from his salary, leaves Bill with $14 per month. Not only is this considerably less than Bill earns in the day activity program, but he must work longer hours to receive it. This is the second job placement for Bill. On the last job he became unhappy over his lack of money and his job performance deteriorated. He was fired and returned to the day activity program where he was "rehabilitated" to his present level again!! How can we help Bill by providing incentives to work?

Answer to Exercise

1-1.   Although the basic problem of wages versus benefits is something you can't change, think about other reinforcers that might help maintain Bill in the community.

Recently some people have recommended attempts be made to reduce the reactivity of the service delivery system for developmentally disabled individuals. Most of these recommendations have focused on prevention (Herbert, 1977; Uitti, 1977; Litch, 1978; Johnson, 1980). There is also a need to reduce the reactivity of the delivery of habilitation services. Lent (1978) and Ziarnik (1980) have suggested that individual programs for clients must begin to emphasize the skills clients need for success, rather than focusing on their deficits or their weaknesses. Direct services would then adopt a proactive model as opposed to one that is reactive. When examining a total service system, we must not overlook the fact that people deliver services, and ideally these people ought to reflect the proactive orientation of the total system. Therefore, as Lent (1978) suggested, reorientation efforts need to be extended to the point of service delivery where proactive staff work with clients.

THE CONCEPT

What exactly does it mean to be proactive when working with a client? *Webster's New Collegiate Dictionary* (1977) defines reactive as "acting in response or opposition to some former state or act," and defines proactive as "involving modification by a factor which precedes that which is modified." Perhaps we can gain a sense of how the two words contrast by comparing words with similar prefixes. While the prefix "re" can carry positive meanings, it is also found in words such as "repeal," which means to cancel or abolish, "reluctant," which involves doing something under protest, or "refract," which means to bias or twist things. The prefix "pro" is found in words such as "progress," which means move onward, "process," which means method, and "produce," which means construct.

When we look at reactive staff-client interactions, we see a lack of planning and an emphasis on responding to a client's behavior after it has begun. The net result is a lowered capacity to develop in the client those behaviors that are necessary for independence outside the agency. Although there is nothing absolutely incorrect about responding to a client's behavior after it has begun, the danger here is similar to the dangers described earlier in the reactive health system or insurance program. We often spend so much time reacting that we don't build positive programs. When staff behavior is entirely reactive, it is costly, inefficient, and self-perpetuating. For example, a program designed to punish aggressive behavior is reactive, because such a program does not necessarily teach the client adaptive behavior. The client may decrease his or her amount of aggressive behavior, but does not learn what to do instead. However, a program that teaches aggressive clients nonviolent alternative means of expressing their feelings is proactive, because it seeks to promote long-term solutions to the problems.

The proactive trainer is really the eternal optimist. He or she views the cup as being "half full" as opposed to being "half empty." How does this translate into client goals? Some examples are:

Reactive Goals	vs.	*Proactive Goals*
Reduce aggression		Teach social skills (nonviolent; assertive)
Decrease leaving work area		Increase on-task time
Stop screaming		Increase quiet time
Stop smelling so badly		Increase personal hygiene

PROACTIVE CHARACTERISTICS

We have been able to identify six major characteristics of a proactive staff person:

1. The proactive staff person knows the client's history.
2. The proactive staff person knows the client presently.
3. The proactive staff person thinks about the client in the future.
4. The proactive staff person knows the agency.
5. The proactive staff person is a professional, not an employee.
6. The proactive staff person works with and for the client.

The following discussions are intended to serve as guidelines to help you become more proactive in your interactions with clients. How many of these fit you and your colleagues?

The Past

The proactive staff person knows the client's history. It is important that staff become as familiar as possible with the social, medical, psychological, and treatment history of the client. This includes past programming successes and failures. A solid understanding of a client's history allows for better judgments about particular program priorities and needs. Without a working knowledge of a client's history, staff are bound to repeat past errors, make judgments in isolation rather than from a broad perspective, and determine programs without knowledge of what has or has not worked in the past. Consider the following example:

Frieda came to the group home after her father died. Her mother was older, and lived in a small town several hours from Happy Homes, Inc. After a few weeks of observation and assessment the staff had a planning meeting. It was noted that, in addition to other problems, Frieda rarely had her shoes tied, and would often extend her untied shoe to a staff member. The team decided to teach Frieda to tie her shoes. Months later, when Frieda's mom came to visit, the staff happily announced that Frieda could now tie her own shoes. Dumbfounded, the mother said "She always could. . . ."

Unfortunately, in present practice, it is often the direct care staff who have the least knowledge of a client's history. In fact, some programs do not allow direct care staff to read the client's "confidential" file. In addition to the negative effects this can have on client programs, denying staff access to files communicates that they are not professionals, are not responsible, and are not to be trusted. In this atmosphere, is it any wonder that direct care staff often feel they are the last consideration in providing services to the client?

The Present

The proactive staff person knows the client presently. To know the client presently, staff must not only be familiar with the client's present needs (which can only follow from a knowledge of history) but must also be totally knowledgeable about present goals, methods of achieving these goals, and progress toward the goals. This knowledge must be updated on a daily basis for clients with whom staff are in daily contact. This increases the consistency that is so essential for successful treatment. Consistency is critical, particularly in programs designed to reduce the occurrence of objectionable or inappropriate behaviors. Objectionable or inappropriate behaviors are not "innate" aspects of developmentally disabled persons. They are not behaviors that a person is born with. Rather, most behaviors that staff find objectionable have developed as a result of learning during interactions with the environment (Rosen, Clark, & Kivitz, 1977). Often it is staff reactions that maintain the client's inappropriate behavior (Bouliew, 1971; Spradlin & Girardeau, 1966).

Unless staff achieve maximum consistency, objectionable behaviors will be maintained by the very environmental consequences that helped originally develop them. Inconsistent use of either reinforcement or punishment has the effect of making a behavior much stronger and more resistant to change. In the case discussed below, it seems that some staff found a client's remarks humorous while others found them objectionable. Just like any comedian on stage, this client's behavior will continue as long as some staff find it funny and laugh. Maximum consistency can only be achieved when individual staff have knowledge of client programs and are in agreement as to how those programs shall be carried out.

Exercise

1-2. The staff were listing a client's strengths and needs during the goal planning session. The needs were all in the area of social behavior. In sum, the client sought attention by making obscene remarks to staff and clients. Despite several months of efforts, the case manager had been unsuccessful in attempts to reduce this behavior. When it came time to list the client's strengths, the first staff person volunteered that the client had "a good sense of humor." Remember, behavior is no mystery; it always gives feedback regarding the environmental consequences that help maintain it.
  1. What might be maintaining the client's objectionable behavior?
  2. What would a proactive staff person do about it?

Answers to Exercises

1-1. 1. If you first thought of social reinforcers based on staff's varying perceptions of "what's funny," you're on the way to becoming proactive.
  2. One of the first things that needs to happen is to get agreement among staff as to what was acceptable and what was objectionable in the client's behavior.

The Future

The proactive staff person thinks about the client in the future. The point of the whole proactive concept is to reduce short-sighted staff-client interactions and to help staff develop holistic approaches to client services. The proactive concept views the client as having a past, a present, and a future, all of which are directly related to programming. Community-based services are in existence because it is hoped that a client's integration into the community will be more likely to occur if training is done in the community, as opposed to training being done in an isolated institution. To meet the habilitation goals of programs for the developmentally disabled, we must avoid making all programs into long-term care facilities. If the client is conceived of as having a future with well-operationalized long-range goals, the focus remains on training and habilitation. It is all too easy to be caught up in day-to-day operations and ignore the future. For example, in programs that rely heavily on client production for fiscal support, the long-range goals of the individual client may receive secondary attention. Since the organization needs profits to employ staff, it becomes easy to focus on furniture stripping, electronics assembly, or envelope stuffing as the important aspects of a client's program. However, no client has ever been placed in a habilitation program because of an inability to strip furniture, assemble electronic components, or stuff envelopes; therefore, production is never an appropriate habilitation goal. *Production is the result of good training, but, in and of itself, production is never training*. To avoid this short-sighted trap, staff are encouraged to ask three questions to help gain a perspective on the client's future:

1. Why is the client here?
2. What is keeping him or her here?

3. How does the present activity help the client overcome the answers to questions one and two?

By constantly questioning the relationship of a given activity to training and goals, community-based programs can begin to fulfill the promised mission of habilitation. And problems like those in the following example can be avoided.

> In the mid 1960s two researchers, Robert Rosenthal and Lenore Jacobson, tested the "self-fulfilling prophecy" in an elementary school classroom (Rosenthal & Jacobson, 1968). They took all the students in several classrooms and pretended to test them. They randomly chose 20% of the students in each class and told the teachers that these children had the greatest potential (remember, they may or may not have had the potential). At the end of the year they checked with the teachers and, sure enough, the teachers rated the randomly labeled students as more appealing, more affectionate, and better adjusted. Just the teachers' expectations were enough for them to view the children as different.

The Agency

The proactive staff person knows the agency. Programs serving the developmentally disabled often attempt to meet too many broad social goals at once (Gettings, 1979). The end result of such attempts is often that none of the goals are met. Given funding levels, number of staff available, and skill levels of most in-house staff, it is virtually impossible for any one facility to be all things to all of its clients. Thus, direct care staff must know the goals of the agency, as well as the limits of the agency. If client needs that are outside the goals of the agency are identified, direct care staff must be familiar with other resources that can best meet these needs.

Consider the following:

> In our professional activities we constantly encounter day activity programs with a staff of 8 or 10. The director of the program has a master's degree in speech pathology, the case manager has a college degree in education and the rest of the staff either have degrees in fields like history or philosophy or have high school diplomas. The agency's stated goal is to "provide for the total habilitation needs of the client." HOW CAN THIS BE? Where are the physicians, psychologists, occupational therapists, or experts in rehabilitation on the staff? Only with such staff can the *total* needs be met. Know your limits and set realistic goals.

Professionalization

The proactive staff person is a professional, not an employee. One thing that direct care staff discover very quickly upon gaining employment in a facility that serves developmentally disabled persons is that they have a major programmatic responsibility, but do not have very high status within the organization. Highest status within the organization is generally given to "professionals." Professionals are persons who have advanced degrees, such as a master's, a doctorate, or an R.N. Although professionals can have considerable knowledge about programs and methods for client treatment, communication with direct care staff is sometimes unclear or couched in terms that only the professional understands.

Professionalization is an issue currently receiving attention from those involved in personnel development programs (Bernstein, 1979). The issue is that professionals need to distribute their skills and knowledge, as well as taking the mystery out of having an advanced degree. This is based on the premise that, with adequate preparation, direct care staff can develop treatment skills equal to that of the professional. The proactive concept suggests that programs achieve maximum effectiveness when direct care staff think of themselves as, and are treated as, professionals. Direct care staff are critical to the success of habilitation programs and cannot be treated as "9 to 5" employees. Thus, the proactive staff person thinks of himself or herself as a technical expert or at least as a potential expert. The proactive staff person not only welcomes supervision and then applies suggestions but also seeks new technical information by reading journals and reports. Further, decisions regarding the client are based on long-term client needs and technical efficiency, not on emotions or short-term gains. Finally, proactive professionals make decisions and follow through on those decisions while holding themselves, others, and clients accountable for their behavior. When proactive staff say they are going to do something, they do it!

Professionalization of direct care staff makes sense from an administrative point of view as well. It is not unusual for direct care staff to have an annual turnover rate ranging between 10% and 50%. Staff turnover is very costly to any organization, but, when it is this high, reduction of staff turnover becomes absolutely necessary. What does professionalization of direct care staff have to do with reducing turnover? Several studies on what motivates people (Herzberg, 1966; Lawler, 1973) suggest that the top reasons for job satisfaction are a sense of achievement and being recognized for work done well. These would be attainable through a staff development program that seeks to professionalize direct care staff. Although programs serving handicapped persons often offer fewer financial benefits than other types of employment, these same studies indicate that, when other factors are equal, salary ranks low as an important reason for staying or not staying on the job.

Client-Centered Orientation

The proactive staff person works with and for the client. This characteristic of proactive staff provides a quite different picture than the one of staff-client relationships held by many people in the field. Often a staff person is seen as a caretaker (they need our help), nondirective (if the barriers to development are removed, development automatically occurs), directive (the clients are happier in routine, controlled environments), or a martyr (you must have so much patience). Although persons may decide to seek employment in facilities serving the developmentally disabled for many reasons, they must never lose sight of the primary goal of employment: habilitation of the client. Toward this end, the proactive staff person treats the client with respect and at the same time follows through on program priorities.

It has been demonstrated many times that people have a large influence on the behavior of others, and that expectations alone can change peoples' behavior. Simply stated, this means if you expect people to be bright, the chances are that they will behave as if they are bright. Similarly, if you expect people to be retarded they will oftentimes meet your expectations by acting retarded. This phenomenon has been called the "self-fulfilling prophecy," or the Pygmalion effect (Merton, 1968). The most widely recognized example is in the play *My Fair Lady*, where a poor uneducated girl was taught to act like a duchess, with the result that everyone thought she was a duchess. Our clients often become what we expect them to become. Although treating a client with respect is not the only thing that will help the client develop respectable behavior, it is necessary for such behavior to develop.

Exercise

1-3. Staff report that Darrel has such a short attention span that he works for only five seconds at a time before losing interest. When you observe him, you notice that, after five seconds of attention to a task, he stops and looks around until he catches the eye of the trainer, who then approaches Darrel, pats him on the back, and tells him to keep working.
   1. Is the trainer proactive?
   2. Why does Darrell work for only five seconds?
   3. What would you do to change Darrel's behavior?

Answers to Exercise

1-3. 1. It is unlikely that the trainer in this example is proactive. A proactive trainer would be likely to pat Darrel on the back when he is working, not when he stops and is looking around.
   2. It is likely that Darrel works for only five seconds at a time because he receives attention from staff only when he stops working. Too many times this is the case. As long as clients are working and quiet, staff are often reluctant to "rock the boat."
   3. To change Darrel's behavior, staff should reinforce him when he's working.

CONCLUSION

Human service systems can no longer afford to remain totally reactive; they must develop holistic approaches that have the capacity both to respond to problems and to prevent their occurrence. Similarly, staff delivering services must develop a holistic approach.

When reading the behavior change literature, one gets the impression that program success is often based upon the "simple" application of a variety of principles and procedures. In the remainder of this book, we attempt to teach a system of analyzing behavior as opposed to specific techniques for behavior change. Although professionals know that you cannot just apply principles or techniques to get change, the cold, austere nature of many behavior change journals and reports can communicate this expectation to novices. In reality, a good deal of preparation and decision-making must occur prior to the selection of any treatment program. Unfortunately, this is rarely communicated in the literature. The qualitative aspects of program implementation, such as how and with what style social reinforcers should be delivered, are also rarely mentioned. To say "social reinforcement is needed" is one thing, but to actually teach someone how to deliver it is another matter. Furthermore the holistic nature of any program receives little written attention. For instance, change in one behavior has the potential to affect other client behaviors. The proactive concept speaks to these "other" considerations that must be taken into account in any client program. These "other" considerations often spell the difference between success and failure of client programming.

SUGGESTED ACTIVITIES

1. Ask another staff person to watch you work with clients for a short period of time (15-20 minutes). Have them count the number of times you praise or otherwise reinforce positive behavior in your clients. No matter what their total count is, try to increase it. Try to catch somebody doing something right!!!
2. Does your facility have an agreed upon list of appropriate social behaviors for clients? If not, get staff together and construct one. It will help promote the consistency needed to increase appropriate client behavior.
3. How many goals for the clients you work with directly can you name? You should be able to name goals for all your clients.
4. How many client goals are written in such a way as to stress increasing behaviors rather than decreasing behaviors? A proactive trainer writes goals to teach clients new skills, not just to eliminate inappropriate behavior.
5. What is the stated purpose of your agency? Of your program within the agency? It is realistic? Ask other staff. How many staff independently agree as to the goal?
6. Observe training in your facility and identify examples of proactive training and examples of reactive training.

REFERENCES

Bernstein, G. S. Behavior analysis, professionalization, and deprofessionalization: Issues and implications. *The Behavior Therapist,* 1979, *2,* 25.
Bernstein, G. S., & Karan, O. Obstacles to vocational normalization for the developmentally disabled. *Rehabilitation Literature,* 1979, *40,* 66-71.

Bouliew, D. Do institutions maintain retarded behavior? *Mental Retardation,* 1971, *9,* 36–38.

Drash, P. W., Boyd, L. A., & Stolberg, A. L. *Prevention of mental retardation and other developmental disabilities: Organizing a national forum.* Presented at the meeting of the American Association on Mental Deficiency, Miami Beach, May, 1979.

Gettings, R. Services to the developmentally disabled: A Washington perspective. In J. P. Ziarnik (Ed.), *Governor's conference on developmental disabilities.* Vermillion: University of South Dakota, 1979.

Herbert, H. J. *Invited address.* Presented to the California Association of Retarded Citizens Agenda for Action Workshop, Sacramento, November, 1977.

Herzberg, F. *Work and the nature of man.* Cleveland: World Publishing Co., 1966.

Houts, P. S., & Scott, R. A. *How to catch your staff doing something right.* Department of Behavioral Science, Pennsylvania State University College of Medicine, 1975.

Johnson, V. P. Prevention of mental retardation. In R. Wynn (Ed.), *Obstetrics and gynecology annual.* Appleton-Century-Crofts, 1980.

Krishef, C. *Characteristics of the service delivery systems on a state and local level.* Presented at the meeting of the American Association on Mental Deficiency, Denver, June, 1978.

Lawler, E. E. *Motivation in work organizations.* Monterey, Calif.: Brooks/Cole Publishing Co., 1973.

Lent, J. R. Organizing service delivery for the severely retarded: A futurist's view. In M. S. Berkler, G. H. Bible, S. M. Boles, D. E. Deitz, & A. C. Ress (Eds.), *Current trends for the developmentally disabled.* Baltimore: University Park Press, 1978.

Litch, S. *Towards prevention of mental retardation in the next generation.* Ft. Wayne, Ind.: Ft. Wayne Printing Co., 1978.

Magrab, P. R., & Elder, J. O. *Planning for services to handicapped persons: Community, education, health.* Baltimore: Paul H. Brookes Publishing Co., 1979.

Merton, R. K. The self-fulfilling prophecy. In R. K. Merton (Ed.), *Social theory and social structure.* New York: The Free Press, 1968.

Rosen, M., Clark, G., & Kivitz, M. S. *Habilitation of the handicapped.* Baltimore: University Park Press, 1977.

Rosenthal, R., & Jacobson, L. *Pygmalion in the classroom.* New York: Holt, Rinehart & Winston, 1968.

Spradlin, J. E., & Girardeau, F. L. The behavior of moderately and severely retarded persons. In N. R. Ellis (Ed.), *International review of research in mental retardation* (Vol. 1). New York: Academic Press, 1966.

Uitti, J. *Prevention: An agenda for action.* Sacramento: California Association for the Retarded, 1977.

Ziarnik, J. Developing proactive direct care staff. *Mental Retardation,* 1980, *18*(6), 289–292.

Chapter 2

Overview of Developmental Disabilities

OBJECTIVES

To be able to:

1. Identify the principal indicators of developmental disabilities (as established by Public Law (PL) 95-602).
2. Describe what is meant by adaptive behavior.
3. Identify one key court case that supports developmentally disabled individuals' rights to treatment, education, and compensation.
4. Identify three principal federal laws that influenced the treatment of developmentally disabled individuals.
5. State the 1977 American Association on Mental Deficiency's (AAMD) definition of mental retardation and list five causes of mental retardation.
6. Define epilepsy and list five causes of epilepsy.
7. Describe the four major classifications of epilepsy.
8. Describe the six types of cerebral palsy and list five causes of cerebral palsy.
9. List five symptoms of autism.

DEVELOPMENTAL DISABILITIES DEFINED

What are developmental disabilities? This apparently simple question seems to call for a brief definition similar to the definitions used in the natural sciences. However, in the area of human services and particularly in the field of developmental disabilities, fundamental concepts regarding what constitute disabilities are not as clear as we would like them to be. As a result, defining developmental disabilities becomes a difficult task.

Recently, Congress has made several attempts to provide a legal definition of developmental disabilities. A legal definition is necessary for allocating public funds for training facilities and educational programs, and for securing the rights of developmentally disabled individuals. The most recent definition, put forth by the 95th Congress in PL 95-602, reads:

> The term developmental disability means a severe, chronic disability of a person that:
>
> A. Is attributable to a mental or physical impairment or combination of mental and physical impairments.
> B. Is manifested before the person attains age 22.
> C. Is likely to continue indefinitely.
> D. Results in substantial functional limitation in three or more of the following areas of major life activity:
>   1. self-care
>   2. receptive and expressive language
>   3. learning
>   4. mobility
>   5. self-direction
>   6. capacity for independent living
>   7. economic self-sufficiency
> E. Reflects the person's need for a combination and sequence of special, inter-disciplinary, or generic care, treatment, or other services that are of lifelong or extended duration and are individually planned and coordinated.

This legal definition of developmental disabilities leaves much room for subjective interpretation. Whereas most human problems, diseases, or disorders are defined by a specific set of characteristic symptoms (i.e., fever and nausea are associated with the flu, or swollen glands with the mumps), developmental disabilities involve deficits in adaptive behavior. Adaptive behavior refers to an individual's ability to meet society's standards of independence and responsibility expected for his or her age (Ingalls, 1978). Perhaps in no other area of human services are the traditional concepts of normalcy and deviancy so apparent, but so challenged, as in the field of developmental disabilities.

If we define developmental disabilities as deficits in adaptive behavior, we are still left with the task of defining what adaptive or maladaptive behaviors are. This is not an easy task, because adaptive behaviors change over time, location, and culture.

Imagine a person standing on a street corner beating himself with a whip. What would happen? Most likely the police would be called to the scene to escort the person to a treatment facility. In fourteenth century Europe, however, when the bubonic plague was killing thousands of people, standing in the street whipping oneself for the sins of mankind was a socially accepted behavior that was not viewed as deviant or maladaptive.

Today, in the United States, there continue to be regional and cultural differences as to what behaviors are considered normal or adaptive. Take for example, a guest at a gala grand opening in New York, dressed in the latest fashions. Although perfectly adaptive at this special occasion, this person's dress would be considered maladaptive if he or she were attending a cattle auction. On the other hand, a farming couple in work clothes would also be considered maladaptive at the Metropolitan Opera.

Similarly, society's attitudes toward developmentally disabled persons have changed over time and place and have resulted in tremendous differences in the care, treatment, and training of developmentally disabled individuals.

HISTORICAL TREATMENT

In the past, the treatment and training of developmentally disabled persons was generally not very humane and was characterized by isolation, abuse, institutionalization, and euthanasia. Ancient Greeks believed that the laws of nature dictated that only the fittest survived; therefore, they abandoned or killed anyone who was handicapped. During medieval times, treatment of developmentally disabled persons varied greatly. Some people treated them as innocent children, while others tolerated them as fools. Still others believed that developmentally disabled individuals were able to communicate with the supernatural or have revelations from God. On the other hand, many individuals were burned at the stake as "witches" because their behavior deviated from society's norms and was thought to be caused by Satan. Both Martin Luther and John Calvin, for example, denounced mentally retarded persons as being possessed by the devil (MacMillan, 1977).

In modern times, even though concern for the developmentally disabled had increased, treatment continued to fall short of the ideal. Blatt (1970) made the following observation:

> Most dayrooms have a series of bleacherlike benches on which sit denuded residents, jammed together, without purposeful activity or communication or any type of interaction. In each dayroom is an attendant or two, whose main function seems to be to "stand around" and, on occasion, hose down the floor, driving excretions into a sewer conveniently located in the center of the room. (p. 17)

Other deplorable conditions were noted by the President's Committee on Mental Retardation:

> The seclusion rooms are small cells with locked doors, barred windows, and are just large enough for one bed and a mattress on the floor. Residents are locked in these rooms without supervision and for long periods of time.
>
> One resident who was recently observed in a seclusion room had been there as long as the ward attendant had been assigned to that ward, which was six years. Physical restraints, including straight jackets, nylon stockings, and rags as well as rope, are often used without physician's orders. One young girl was observed in a straight jacket, tied to a wooden bench. It was explained that she sucked her fingers and had been so restrained for nine years. (1973, p. 24)

In addition, educational programming was neglected. Thormahlen (1965) recorded the daily routine of direct care staff in an institution. Only 12% of the total time was spent in activities and programs that promoted independent behaviors of the residents. Furthermore, less than 2% of the direct care staff's time was spent in formal teaching sessions.

Today, a variety of new programs have been developed in order to improve the quality of care, training, and treatment of developmentally disabled persons. One of the more recent and progressive of these programs is the establishment of community-based training facilities. These programs are the result of advances in behavioral treatment techniques, advocates on behalf of the developmentally disabled, legislative mandates, and legal decisions.

Exercises

2-1.   Mary Johnson, age 32, was referred to your facility. Upon assessment it was found that she had suffered from polio at age 12, which left her legs permanently paralyzed. With prosthetic aids (i.e., braces) she is able to function well on her own in her home. Mary has no apparent intellectual deficiencies. Under PL 95-602, would Mary be considered developmentally disabled? Why?

2-2.   Adaptive behavior refers to the ability of an individual to _____

Answers to Exercises

2-1.   No. Mary does not exhibit substantial limitations in the areas of self-care, receptive and expressive language, learning, self-direction, capacity for independent living, or economic self-sufficiency.

2-2.   Adaptive behavior refers to the ability of an individual to meet society's standards of independence and responsibility expected for his or her age.

LEGAL ISSUES

How did the education and treatment of developmentally disabled persons become a legal issue?

In the past, most courts refrained from investigating the care or treatment of the handicapped. Generally, developmentally disabled persons were viewed as second-class citizens who were not entitled to all of the legal rights and privileges of other citizens. Furthermore, the courts felt that treatment decisions were similar to medical decisions, and therefore should be left up to the experts. Lately, however, the courts have passed decisions based on the federal constitution that have guaranteed developmentally disabled individuals the same constitutional rights enjoyed by all citizens. In particular, these rights include the right to education, the right to treatment, and the right to compensation for work.

Right to Education

The major court cases regarding the right to education were *Brown v. Board of Education of Topeka, Kansas* (1954), *Pennsylvania Association for Retarded Children (PARC) v. Commonwealth of Pennsylvania* (1972), and *Mills v. Board of Education of District of Columbia* (1972).

The primary focus of the *Brown v. Board of Education of Topeka, Kansas* (1954) decision by the United States Supreme Court was that racial segregation, prevalent in American school systems at the time, was unconstitutional. The importance of this case for developmentally disabled persons, however, was the Court's opinion that education is good for everyone, tends to awaken children to our cultural values, and helps them to adjust normally to the environment.

Later, in a related case (*Wolf v. the State of Utah,* 1969), two mentally retarded children were excluded from school because the school could not provide programming for children with these disabilities. The court ruled that education was a fundamental and inalienable right guaranteed by the United States Constitution. This ruling made education mandatory for all children in the state of Utah, regardless of their level of intellectual functioning.

One of the more notable cases regarding the right to education for the developmentally disabled was the *Pennsylvania Association for Retarded Children (PARC) v. Commonwealth of Pennsylvania* (1972). Before 1972 thousands of children were denied educational services under a Pennsylvania state law that specified that children who were viewed as being unable to benefit from education could be excluded from school. The major court decisions in this case included the following:

1. All children, regardless of the degree of disability, can benefit from a program of education and training.
2. All developmentally disabled children are entitled to *free* access to a public program of education and training.
3. Placement in educational settings should be appropriate to the child's abilities, with placement in a regular classroom preferable to a special classroom, and a special classroom preferable to any type of institutional placement.
4. Change in educational placements must comply with a due process hearing procedure.
5. Periodic 2-year reevaluations of a child's educational placement are required.

In a further extension of the decision resulting from the *PARC* case, the courts ruled in *Mills v. Board of Education of the District of Columbia* (1972) that all children, regardless of their disabilities or behavioral symptoms, were entitled to free public education. In addition, the court ruled that a lack of funds was an insufficient reason for not providing educational programs to these citizens.

In summary, the federal and state courts have found that the right to free and appropriate education is a constitutionally guaranteed right. Furthermore, this right cannot be denied because of a person's level of adaptive behavior or because of expenses incurred by the schools in providing the educational program.

Right to Treatment

The hallmark case on the right to treatment was *Wyatt v. Stickney* (1971). In the early 1970s, staff reductions were ordered in Alabama's residential facilities serving developmentally disabled persons. These staff reductions were required because of state budgetary cutbacks. A lawsuit was then brought against the institutions on behalf of the residents. In this case the court concluded that Alabama's entire mental health and mental retardation system was constitutionally inadequate. The court expressed the opinion that the residents of state facilities had every right to receive adequate treatment so that they could return to the community as soon as possible.

Specific findings were that Partlow State School and Hospital for the Mentally Retarded was a "warehousing" institution with an inhumane psychological and physical environment, incapable of providing treatment and rehabilitation. Deficiencies noted at Partlow included the absence of individualized treatment plans, unqualified staff in numbers insufficient to administer adequate treatment, and the requirement that residents perform nontherapeutic uncompensated work. To correct these and other deficiencies the court ordered the hiring of 300 additional employees within 30 days, the review of all medication programs by a team of physicians, and the formation of a human rights committee to ensure the dignity and human rights of the residents. It should be noted that, although the legal action specifically addressed Partlow State School, the ruling has implications for all state, public, and private agencies serving developmentally disabled individuals.

In addition to ensuring adequate staff and protection of constitutional rights, federal courts have also awarded monetary damages to patients because of an institution's failure to provide adequate treatment, as in the case of *Donaldson v. O'Conner* (1974). Mr. Donaldson was committed to a Florida mental institution and refused, for religious reasons, the two therapies (i.e., electroshock and tranquilizing drugs) presented to him. Because of this refusal, Mr. Donaldson was not offered any alternative therapy for the next 15 years. As a result, Mr. Donaldson sued for damages and was awarded $38,500, which was assessed against the superintendent and staff psychiatrist.

Right to Compensation

Another area of judicial concern is the right to compensation for institution-maintaining labor. The case of *Souder v. Brennan* (1973) had a major impact in this area. Eugene Souder had been institutionalized for over 30 years. He worked in the institution kitchen approximately 11 hours per day, seven days a week. For his work, Souder was reimbursed $2.00 per month and received two days off each month. The conclusion of the court was that not all work assignments are therapeutic in nature and that the Thirteenth Amendment forbids slavery and involuntary servitude. The court ruled that when work assignments are for institutional maintenance, rather than for therapeutic goals, the minimum wage must be paid to the institutional resident.

In summary, United States courts have acted to protect developmentally disabled individuals and their constitutional rights. The courts have ruled that developmentally disabled persons are entitled to all the constitutional rights of every citizen and have specifically identified the following rights:

1. The Right to Education
2. The Right to Treatment
3. The Right to Compensation

Exercises

2-3. List the major court cases pertaining to the Right to Education, the Right to Treatment, and the Right to Compensation.

2-4. The *PARC v. Commonwealth of Pennsylvania* decision established which of the following educational rights of developmentally disabled persons?
   a. All developmentally disabled individuals can benefit from education.
   b. Public education and training programs for developmentally disabled persons must be free of charge.
   c. Developmentally disabled individuals are entitled to periodic evaluations of their educational placements.
   d. Change in educational placements must comply with a due process hearing procedure.
   e. Placements of developmentally disabled individuals in regular or special education classrooms are preferable to any kind of institutional placement.
   f. All of the above.

2-5. The *Mills v. Board of Education (District of Columbia)* decision guaranteed free public education for all handicapped children, but, at the same time, stated that a state may be excused from providing educational services for developmentally disabled children in cases where the state budget could not afford it.
   True _____ False _____

2-6. The *Brown v. Board of Education* decision stated that:
   a. Schools without special programs for developmentally disabled children are in violation of the constitution.
   b. Education is good for everyone.

c. Education is necessary for teaching basic academic skills but should not attempt to teach cultural values.
d. Education is an important factor for the normal adjustment of children to society.
e. b and d.

2-7. In the *Donaldson v. O'Conner* (1974) case, the superintendent and staff psychiatrist at the Florida State Hospital were sued for:
a. Using electroshock for therapy.
b. Using tranquilizing drugs as therapy.
c. Not providing treatment to a patient.
d. a and b.

2-8. In *Souder v. Brennan* (1973), the court ruled that:
a. Institutionalized developmentally disabled individuals are not allowed to work.
b. Every type of work performed by institutionalized individuals must be compensated according to the prevalent minimum wage standards.
c. All nontherapeutic labor performed by institutionalized residents must be compensated at the minimum wage.
d. It is reasonable to expect free institution-maintaining work from all capable institutional residents.

Answers to Exercises

2-3. Right to Education:
Brown v. Board of Education of Topeka, Kansas (1954)
Wolf v. State of Utah (1969)
Pennsylvania Association for Retarded Children v. Commonwealth of Pennsylvania (1972)
Mills v. Board of Education of District of Columbia (1972)
Right to Treatment:
Wyatt v. Stickney (1971)
Donaldson v. O'Conner (1974)
Right to Compensation:
Souder v. Brennan (1973)

2-4. f
2-5. False
2-6. e
2-7. c
2-8. c

Federal Legislation

Congress has also expressed concern for the rights of developmentally disabled persons. In 1970, Congress passed the first federal Developmental Disabilities Act, PL 91-517. This law provided the first legal definition of a developmental disability as a disability that was attributable to mental retardation, cerebral palsy, epilepsy, or other neurological conditions closely related to mental retardation. The disability must occur between birth and 18 years of age and constitute a substantial handicap to the individual. This definition was later expanded by the 94th Congress in PL 94-103 to include autism. In addition, the 94th Congress passed PL 94-142, which provided the critical definition of the rights of all developmentally disabled children. The basic rights established by PL 94-142 included:

1. *The right to due process,* protecting children from erroneous classification, labeling, and denial of equal educational opportunities.
2. *Protection against discriminatory testing and diagnosis* by using unbiased or culture-free intelligence tests.
3. *The right to an education* in the least restrictive environment.
4. *The right to individualized program plans* ensuring quality and accountability by those individuals responsible for the education of handicapped children.

Additionally, minimum standards for Individualized Program Plans (IPPs) were set by PL 94-142. An adequate IPP is required to meet the following criteria:

1. It must be developed by a joint conference, including care providers, the client, and the client's guardian, and must be presented in writing.
2. It should include specific descriptions of the client's conditions and needs.
3. It should specify intermediate and long-term treatment goals.
4. It should include a timetable for expected goal attainment.
5. All services to be provided should be listed in detail.
6. Service delivery agencies and treatment personnel should be indicated.
7. It should specify how the services can be provided in the normal or least restrictive environment.
8. It should state objective criteria for treatment evaluation procedures, and should list schedules for evaluations.
9. It should be reviewed periodically.

Summary of Federal Legislation and Court Decisions

As you can see, the care and treatment of developmentally disabled persons have changed significantly from medieval times. It seems ironic that many of the changes did not occur until the federal courts and the U.S. Congress intervened. Today many professionals still maintain the attitude that there is no need to be aware of these recent legal decisions. The Supreme Court, however, expressed a very different view in the case of *Wood v. Stricklaw* (1975). In this case, the Supreme Court dealt with the school board's failure to observe the constitutional rights of some of its students.

In its own defense, the school board maintained that they did not know they were not following the law, and that they were immune from prosecution because they (the school board) were acting in good faith. However, the Court ruled that operating in a position of responsibility while in ignorance of the constitutional rights of those for whom you care is the same as acting with malice. In such cases, there is no immunity to the law.

In summary, all clients have rights, and you must know the rights of those for whom you care. If you do not know the law and observe it, you may find yourself in violation not only of the law but, more importantly, of the rights of your clients.

CHARACTERISTICS OF DEVELOPMENTAL DISABILITIES

Although PL 95-602 has defined developmental disabilities in terms of deficits in adaptive behavior, there are several types of handicapping conditions that are common among developmentally disabled individuals. These disabilities are mental retardation, epilepsy, cerebral palsy, and autism.

Mental Retardation

When discussing mental retardation, it must be pointed out that there is no universally accepted definition of mental retardation. Professionals from a variety of backgrounds, such as education, psychology, medicine, and rehabilitation, are interested in mental retardation. Each discipline, however, utilizes its own concepts, definitions, and assumptions while providing services to mentally retarded individuals.

In an effort to reduce the differences among professions, the American Association on Mental Defiency (AAMD) proposed the following definition of mental retardation:

> Mental retardation refers to significantly subaverage general intellectual functioning, existing concurrently with deficits in adaptive behavior, which is manifested during the developmental period. (Grossman, 1977, p. 11)

This definition requires that we further define deficits in intellectual ability and adaptive behavior. Intellectual functioning or ability is measured by standardized intelligence tests (IQ tests). The more common are the Stanford-Binet form L-M, the Wechsler Adult Intelligence Scales (WAIS), and the Wechsler Intelligence Scales for Children–Revised (WISC-R). The IQ scores obtained from these tests have a normal curve distribution, with the average IQ score equal to 100, and a standard deviation of approximately 15. What this means is that if you were to administer IQ tests to all individuals in the country, the average IQ score of all these individuals would be 100. Additionally, 64% of all individuals would have IQ scores between 85 and 115. This corresponds to the standard deviation of $\pm$ 15 IQ points. Roughly 95% of all individuals have IQ scores between 70 and 130, or 2 standard deviations ($\pm$ 30 points) above or below 100. To be labeled mentally retarded (significantly subaverage general intellectual functioning), a person must obtain an IQ score more than 2 standard deviations below the average, or approximately an IQ score below 70.

Remember, however, that a low IQ score by itself does not mean that the person can be labeled mentally retarded. The deficit in intellectual functioning must be accompanied by a deficit in adaptive behavior. Adaptive behavior refers to an individual's ability to meet society's standards of independence and responsibility expected for his or her age. Adaptive behaviors refer to a wide range of behaviors that change over time, location, and culture. For example, in determining leisure activities that could be part of a training curriculum, it may be appropriate to teach roller skating if your clients live in an urban area. Roller skating through a rural community that has few sidewalks is not necessarily adaptive.

As you can see, defining adaptive behaviors becomes a difficult task. In attempts to better measure adaptive behavior, a variety of behavioral assessment devices have been developed. Behavioral "checklists" that are available include the AAMD Adaptive Behavior Scale, the Camelot Behavioral Checklist, and the Minnesota Developmental Programming System. These checklists are designed to identify adaptive and maladaptive behaviors that are relatively free of cultural and location influences.

The last part of the AAMD definition of mental retardation indicates that the deficits in adaptive behavior and intellectual functioning must occur during the developmental period. PL 95-602 has defined the developmental period as up to 22 years of age.

As a final note, each state may use its own definition of mental retardation. The more common differences between the AAMD definition and individual state definitions are in the age range considered to be the developmental period and the level of intellectual impairment considered significantly subaverage.

Causes of Mental Retardation There are many causes of mental retardation. However, in one third of all cases of mental retardation, the cause is unknown. Generally speaking, there are two broad categories of mental retardation; one category consists of cases of mental retardation caused by specific organic disorders and the other category consists of cases of mental retardation in which there are no apparent organic causes. These causes may operate before, during, or after birth (MacMillan, 1977; Ingalls, 1978).

Genetic Influence One important cause of mental retardation that operates before birth is genetic influence. A genetically normal individual has 23 pairs of chromosomes (a total of 46 chromosomes) within each cell in his or her body. These pairs of chromosomes are the result of the mother and father each contributing 23 chromosomes to the child. Each chromosome carries genetic information in the form of genes. Thus, genetic information or traits are passed on to the child from the parents.

One type of genetic influence is a sex-linked disorder. Sex-linked disorders are transferred to the child by the sex (X and Y) chromosomes. A female has two X chromosomes and a male has an X and a Y chromosome. Each parent contributes one sex chromosome to the child. The mother always contributes an X chromosome but the father may contribute either an X or a Y. The offspring will have either a female combination (XX) or a male combination (XY). The Y chromosome's principal function is to establish the sex of the child; it does not carry other genetic information. Therefore, if a boy inherits a defective X chromosome from his mother, the disorder associated with the defect will be present, since the Y chromosome carries no other genetic information to counteract the effect of the disorder (see Figure 2-1).

A second type of genetic influence is a mutation. Mutations refer to chromosomes in which new forms of genes develop. Mutations may be caused by radiation, viruses, or chemicals.

A third type of genetic influence occurs when there are abnormal numbers or structures of chromosomes. These are called aberrant chromosomes.

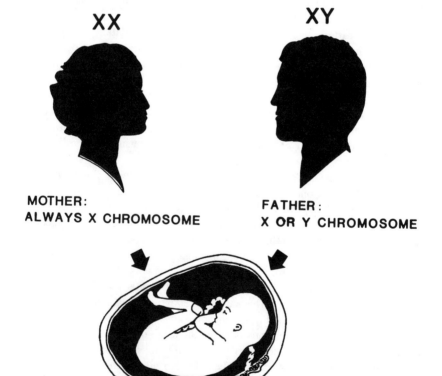

Figure 2-1.   Inheritance of sex-linked disorders.

The most common aberrant chromosome is called a trisomy, which occurs when the cell divides and produces three chromosomes instead of the usual two. Down's syndrome is trisomy 21, which means there are three twenty-first chromosomes rather than two.

Causes Before, During, and After Birth Other causes of mental retardation that may operate before birth include poor maternal diet and nutrition, chronic maternal illness, fetal (infant) malnutrition, and maternal infections such as rubella, syphilis, and other viruses. Additionally, there are many environmental influences that may cause mental retardation. These include ingestion of chemicals, drugs, and alcohol by the mother. As you can see, there are many factors that may lead to mental retardation in the unborn child (fetus). Since the child is a part of the mother, good maternal health is essential during pregnancy.

Mental retardation can also occur during birth, especially with high-risk pregnancies. A pregnancy is considered to be high risk when the mother is under 20 or over 40 years of age, or when the mother has had a history of miscarriages, stillbirths, premature births, previous children with significant birth defects, or other problems. Experiences that affect the child during birth and may cause mental retardation are physical trauma during birth, asphyxia (lack of oxygen), hypoglycemia (low blood sugar levels), or infection.

Causes of mental retardation that operate after birth include infant malnutrition, trauma as a result of injury or accident, infections such as meningitis, drug overdoses, and the ingestion of chemicals such as pesticides and various metals such as lead, arsenic, and mercury. Prolonged fever and illness may also result in mental retardation.

Exercises

2-8. In order to be classified as being mentally retarded, an individual:
   a. Must have a low IQ and exhibit maladaptive behavior.
   b. Must have an IQ of 50, be deficient in adaptive behaviors, and be no older than 18.
   c. Must have subaverage general intellectual functioning, existing concurrently with deficits in adaptive behavior, which is manifested during the developmental period.
   d. Must meet the requirements of PL 95-602.
   e. Must have an IQ of 70, be deficient in adaptive behaviors, and be under 21.
2-9. List five causes of mental retardation.

Answers to Exercises

2-8. c
2-9.

Genetic influence	High-risk pregnancies	Drugs
Toxicity	Poor diet	Alcohol
Infections	Malnutrition	Maternal illness
Anoxia	Hypoglycemia	Trauma

Epilepsy

Epilepsy affects approximately 15 million people in the world (Ward, Jasper, & Pope, 1969) and probably 4 million people in the United States alone (Arangio, 1974). It is one of the more common neurological disorders, and is defined as a sudden disturbance of central nervous system function that is recurrent and is associated with an excessive neuronal discharge that is usually self-limited (Aird & Woodbury, 1974). To better understand this definition, let us examine the brain. The brain is comprised of billions and billions of neurons. Our behaviors, thoughts, and emotions result from the discharges of these neurons. These discharges give off electrical impulses in the form of brain waves from the scalp that can be recorded by an electroencephalograph or EEG. A normal EEG is characterized by low-voltage, fast brain waves. These are called alpha or beta brain waves and are usually 8–16 cycles per second and approximately 25–100 microvolts in amplitude. Epileptic discharges, however, are characterized by low-frequency brain waves (1–3 cycles per second) that are of high voltage. The amplitude of the abnormal brain waves may be greater than 300 microvolts (Schmidt & Wilder, 1968).

The definition of epilepsy as a sudden disturbance of central nervous system function means that the abnormal epileptic discharges occur very suddenly. Usually there is not a gradual disruption of normal EEG activity but rather an instantaneous disruption. That is why most individuals have no warning of when seizures will begin. However, some individuals with epilepsy do have "auras," which are vague sensations indicating that a seizure may be about to occur.

The definition of epilepsy also states that the excessive neuronal discharge is recurrent, meaning that the discharge occurs repeatedly. The discharges are usually self-limited, meaning that the seizures usually stop by themselves.

The major factors influencing the behavioral and clinical manifestations of seizures are the origin and spread of the epileptic discharge in the brain. The discharge may originate in any portion of the brain and the resulting manifestations are related to the particular cortical area involved (see Figure 2-2). For example, Jacksonian epilepsy consists of jerking movements beginning in one joint, such as the thumb, and then gradually spreading to the wrist, elbow, and finally the entire arm. Epileptic seizures with visual symptoms originate in the occipital cortex, the cortical area located at the back of the skull. Visual symptoms reported by individuals include seeing dancing objects, spots, flashes of colors, and a dimming or blurring of vision.

The spread of the discharge over the cortex also has a major influence on behavioral manifestations. The discharge may be limited to a specific cortical location, in which case the behavioral manifestations will be limited to a specific body location, or the discharge may spread over the entire cortex, in which case the behavioral manifestations may involve the entire body.

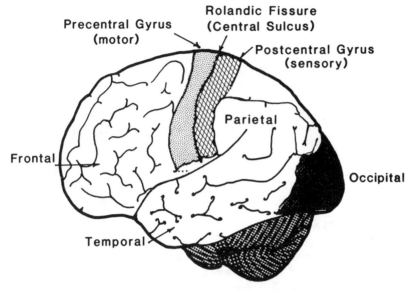

Figure 2-2.   Major divisions of the human cortex.

The International Classification of Epileptic Seizures (Gastaut, 1970) has divided seizures into four major types: partial, unilateral, generalized, and unknown (Table 2-1). In *partial seizures,* the epileptic discharge is limited to a specific site or group of neurons. Partial seizures are sometimes called focal seizures because they involve a specific portion of the body. Partial seizures with psychomotor symptoms originate in the temporal lobe area. Persons afflicted with this type of seizure will often engage in a purposeful behavior at an inappropriate time. For example, a person may begin to smooth his clothing or untie his tie.

In *unilateral seizures* the epileptic discharge is limited to one side of the brain. The resulting behavioral manifestations are limited to the opposite side of the body. For example, in unilateral clonic seizures, a rhythmic jerking motion will occur, but it will involve the limbs on only one side of the body.

Generalized seizures are seizures in which the epileptic discharge spreads over both hemispheres of the brain, and subsequently the seizure may involve the entire body. The two most common types of generalized seizures are absence and tonic-clonic seizures. The main characteristic of an absence seizure, often referred to as a petit mal seizure, is a brief arrest or lapse in consciousness lasting usually only a second or two. The tonic-clonic seizure, or grand mal seizure, consists of two major phases. The tonic phase, which lasts approximately 10–60 seconds, is characterized by the skeletal muscles of the body becoming extremely tense and rigid. Following this the clonic phase begins, in which rhythmic contractions of the body and limbs occur. Uncon-

Table 2–1. International classification of epileptic seizures

Type of Seizure	Common Terminology
I. Partial seizures or seizures beginning locally	
A. Partial seizures with elementary symptomatology (generally without impairment of consciousness)	
1. With motor symptoms	Jacksonian; epilepsia partialis continuans; adversive seizures
2. With special sensory or somatosensory symptoms	Somatosensory seizures; visual auditory seizures
3. With autonomic symptoms	Abdominal epilepsy; epigastric epilepsy
4. Compound forms	
B. Partial seizures with complex symptomatology (generally with impairment of consciousness; may sometimes begin with elementary symptomatology)	Psychomotor or temporal lobe epilepsy
1. With impaired consciousness only	Fugue state
2. With cognitive symptoms	Illusions; dreamy states; déjà vu
3. With affective symptoms	Gelastic seizures
4. With psychosensory symptoms	Olfactory and gustatory hallucinations
5. With psychomotor symptoms	Psychomotor seizures; automatisms
6. Compound forms	
C. Partial seizures secondarily generalized	Tonic, clonic, or grand mal following focal onset
II. Generalized seizures, bilateral symmetrical seizures, or seizures without local onset	
A. Absences	
1. Simple absences with impairment of consciousness only	Petit mal
2. Complex absences, with other phenomena associated with impairment of consciousness	
B. Bilateral massive epileptic myoclonus	Generalized myoclonus; myoclonic jerks
C. Infantile spasms	Infantile spasms
D. Clonic seizures	Clonic seizures; salam seizures; head nodding
E. Tonic seizures	Tonic seizures; brainstem seizures

(continued)

Table 2–1. (*continued*)

Type of Seizure	Common Terminology
F. Tonic-clonic seizures	Grand mal
G. Atonic seizures	
1. Of very brief duration	Drop attacks
2. Of longer duration	Atonic absences; apoplectic epileptic attacks
H. Akinetic seizures	Akinetic seizures
III. Unilateral or predominantly unilateral seizures	Hemiclonic; hemi-motor/ sensory seizures
IV. Unclassified seizures (incomplete data)	

sciousness usually occurs in both phases and the person may lapse into deep sleep following the seizure.

The last type of seizure is categorized as *unknown*. These are seizures in which there is insufficient evidence to classify them into one of the other categories. Since there is a fundamental relationship between the location and spread of the epileptic discharge and its behavioral manifestations, it is essential to provide an accurate description of the seizure so that it may be correctly identified.

Causes of Epilepsy The causes of epilepsy are varied and are similar to the causes of mental retardation. Known causes of epilepsy include lesions in the brain, trauma involving the brain (brain injury resulting from birth trauma, head injuries, hemorrhages in the brain, etc.), brain tumors, cerebrovascular disease, anoxia, hypoglycemia, errors of amino acid metabolism, ingestion of poisons, drug or alcohol withdrawal, elevated body temperatures, infections, and maternal illness. There is also some evidence that genetic factors may result in a predisposition for the development of epilepsy (Schmidt & Wilder, 1968). Some types of seizures appear to be transmitted by dominant genes. However, the actual expression of seizures in offspring varies in relation to the individual's age and other unknown factors. The risk of epilepsy among related individuals decreases with genetic distance.

Pharmacological Treatment The control of seizures in most persons with epilepsy is based upon the regular administration of anticonvulsant medications. However, anticonvulsant medications are not without their problems in terms of treatment effectiveness and reported toxic side effects. Approximately 20% of the epileptic population are unable to control their seizures with these medications. The most common toxic side effects reported include sedation and lethargy. Phenobarbital, a widely used anticonvulsant, has sedative side effects. Dilantin's reported side effects include lethargy, drowsiness, confusion, gum hypertrophy, and hepatitis. Also, there is no universal medication that prevents all types of seizures. Instead different medications are prescribed for different types of seizures.

Exercises

2-9. How is epilepsy defined?
2-10. What are the major factors influencing the behavioral and clinical manifestations of epileptic seizures?
2-11. List and describe the four major types of seizures.
2-12. List five causes of epilepsy.

Answers to Exercises

2-9. Epilepsy is defined as a sudden disturbance of the central nervous system function that is recurrent and is associated with an excessive neuronal discharge that is usually self-limited.
2-10. The site of origin of the epileptic discharge and the spread of the discharge over the cortex.
2-11. Partial seizures are seizures in which the epileptic discharge is limited to a specific site or group of neurons. An example of this type of seizure is the partial seizure with psychomotor symptoms.
    Unilateral seizures are seizures in which the epileptic discharge is limited to one hemisphere of the brain. The resulting behavioral manifestations are limited to the opposite side of the body.
    Generalized seizures are seizures in which the epileptic discharge spreads over both hemispheres of the brain, and subsequently the seizure may involve the entire body. The two most common types of generalized seizures are the absence and tonic-clonic seizures.
    The last type of seizures is categorized as unknown. This is because of the lack of sufficient evidence to classify them into one of the other categories.

2-12.

Genetic influence	High-risk pregnancies	Drugs
Toxicity	Poor diet	Alcohol
Infections	Malnutrition	Maternal illness
Anoxia	Hypoglycemia	Trauma

Cerebral Palsy

Cerebral palsy is a general term that refers to a paralysis, weakness, or incoordination of the motor system (Keats, 1965). It is a permanently disabling condition that results from damage to the central nervous system, and may occur before, during, or after birth. The damage to central nervous system function affects voluntary muscle control, which results in a loss or impairment of control. The extent of involvement varies dramatically, ranging from awkward or involuntary movements to total loss of skeletal muscle control.

    Although cerebral palsy may be classified in several ways, the most common classification is by type. The six main types are spasticity, athetosis, ataxia, tremor, rigidity, and mixed (Keats, 1965; Finnie, 1974).

    In *spasticity,* there is a loss of voluntary muscle control in which coordinated movement becomes extremely difficult. Often the slightest stimulation causes the person to become extremely rigid, and exaggerated reflexes are common. Severe trembling, muscle spasms, and irregular movements may occur. When a deliberate effort to correct or control the incoordination is made, the movements become worse rather than better.

Athetosis or athetoid movement is characterized by constantly recurring, slow, involuntary writhing movements that may affect the limbs of the body. The hands and arms are frequently the most seriously involved. Again, attempts to control these movements often result in increased severity. Involuntary movements often decrease or disappear, however, when the person becomes relaxed or sleeps.

Ataxia is characterized by a disturbance in balance and depth perception, which is reflected in the person's posture and gait. When walking, the person may appear to be dizzy, with awkward movements, staggering, and swaying, and oftentimes speech is slurred.

The *tremor* type of cerebral palsy is characterized by slight tremors similar to those that occur with Parkinsonism, and may involve the entire body or just a part of it.

Rigidity is caused by a disturbance of the extensor and flexor muscles, in which the muscles contract slowly and stiffly. This loss of elasticity of the muscles results in clumsiness.

The last category of cerebral palsy is *mixed,* in which the characteristic involvement is due to two or more of the above categories. For example, a mixed case of spasticity and athetosis is more common than a pure case of either.

The motor impairment resulting from the different types of cerebral palsy may involve all limbs and extremities, only the legs or arms, both limbs on one side of the body, one limb, or only a portion of the limb. The extent of impairment may be so slight that it is unnoticed, or be of such magnitude that the person is extensively handicapped, requiring a wheelchair and assistance with basic self-help skills.

Causes of Cerebral Palsy The causes of cerebral palsy are similar to the causes of mental retardation and epilepsy. They are related to problems that occur before, during, or after birth, such as head trauma, anoxia, toxicity, complications during labor or delivery, or diseases during pregnancy, including syphilis, meningitis, and encephalitis. The cause of more than one third of the cases of cerebral palsy, however, is unknown. The incidence of cerebral palsy is estimated to be one or two cases per 1,000 births.

Autism

Autism refers to a disorder occurring in childhood in which the child is unresponsive to his or her environment. Symptoms of this disorder include:

1. Poorly developed speech or complete absence of speech.
2. Severe withdrawal and lack of the establishment of attachments to other persons.

3. Disturbances of perception, such as overreaction to auditory sounds at some times and total disregard of these sounds at other times.
4. Odd and repetitive use of objects, such as flicking, twirling, and spinning of toys in an inappropriate manner.
5. Stereotypic behaviors such as hand waving, body rocking, and clapping hands.

In the past it was thought that early deprivation of parental love or a combination of environmental and organic factors was responsible for the development of this disorder. Today, although the specific causes are still unknown, autism is thought to be caused by an organic impairment of the central nervous system.

The incidence of autism is estimated to be four to five cases per 10,000 population, with more males than females being affected. Children are usually diagnosed as autistic within the first 3 years of life, but, because of the lack of a clear-cut definition of autism and an overlap of symptoms with other disorders, such as mental retardation and childhood schizophrenia or psychosis, many times these children receive more than one diagnosis.

Exercises

2-13. Define cerebral palsy.
2-14. List and describe the six types of cerebral palsy.
2-15. List five causes of cerebral palsy.
2-16. List five behavioral characteristics of autism.
2-17. Is autism clearly defined?

Answers to Exercises

2-13. Cerebral palsy is a general term that refers to a paralysis, weakness, or incoordination of the motor system.
2-14. Spasticity—In spasticity there is a loss of voluntary muscle control in which coordinated movement becomes extremely difficult. Severe trembling, muscle spasms, and irregular movements may occur.
Athetosis—This type of cerebral palsy is characterized by constantly recurring, slow involuntary writhing movements that may affect the limbs.
Ataxia—Ataxia is characterized by a disturbance in balance and depth perception that affects a person's posture and gait.
Tremor—The tremor type of cerebral palsy is characterized by slight tremors similar to those that occur with Parkinsonism.
Rigidity—Rigidity is caused by a disturbance of the extensor and flexor muscles in which the muscles contract slowly and stiffly.
Mixed—This category refers to cases of cerebral palsy in which the characteristic involvement is due to two or more of the above categories.
2-15. The causes of cerebral palsy are similar to the causes of mental retardation and epilepsy.
2-16. Symptoms of autism include:
1. Poorly developed speech.
2. Lack of attachments to other persons.

3. Disturbances of perception.
4. Odd and repetitive use of objects.
5. Stereotypic behaviors.

2-17. No

SUMMARY

In summary, the term developmental disability refers to a disability that:

1. May be due to mental or physical impairment.
2. Occurs before age 22.
3. Is likely to continue for life.
4. Requires a need for continued services.
5. Results in substantial limitations in three or more of the following areas: a) self-care, b) receptive and expressive language, c) learning, d) mobility, e) self-direction, f) capacity for independent living, and g) economic self-sufficiency.

The more common developmental disabilities are attributable to mental retardation, epilepsy, cerebral palsy, and autism. These disabilities may occur singularly or in combination. However, remember that, even though a person may have one of these conditions, unless there is a substantial deficit in adaptive behavior, the person is not considered to be developmentally disabled.

SUGGESTED ACTIVITIES

1. Obtain a copy of your state's definition of developmental disabilities. Note differences between state and federal definitions.
2. Compare the state definition of mental retardation with the AAMD definition.
3. Has your facility ensured your clients' constitutional rights? If not, what can you do? You should begin by contacting your State Protection and Advocacy Program through your State Office of Developmental Disabilities.
4. List three behaviors or activities that are considered adaptive in your location, but may not be considered adaptive in other settings. Additionally, give three examples of adaptive behaviors that have changed over time.
5. Carefully examine the behaviors of a client in your facility. List five behaviors that are maladaptive. Compare this list of behaviors with the client's goals. Do they coordinate? If not, why not?
6. How many of your clients have epilepsy? What is the International Classification category for each of their diagnoses?
7. List five anticonvulsant medications that your clients receive. Use a Physician's Desk Reference or pharmacology text and list the side effects that may be associated with the use of these medications.
8. Have your public health nurse or an Epilepsy Foundation representative visit your facility and talk about epilepsy and what you can do during a client's seizure.

ADDITIONAL RESOURCES

Begab, M. J. *The mentally retarded and society*. Baltimore: University Park Press, 1975.

Kozloff, M. A. *Reaching the autistic child*. Champaign, Ill.: Research Press, 1977.

Ritvo, E. R. *Autism: Diagnosis, current research and management*. New York: Halsted Press, 1977.

Rosen, M., Clark, G. R., & Kivitz, M. S. *Habilitation of the handicapped*. Baltimore: University Park Press, 1977.

Smith, R. M. *An introduction to mental retardation*. New York: McGraw-Hill, 1971.

Telford, C. W., & Sawrey, J. M. *The exceptional individual*. New Jersey: Prentice-Hall, 1972.

Wood, M. M. *Developmental therapy for young children with autistic characteristics*. Baltimore: University Park Press, 1978.

AUDIOVISUAL MATERIALS

The following audiovisual materials are recommended and may be obtained through: Community Education & Technical Assistance Center, Box C234, John F. Kennedy Child Development Center, University of Colorado Health Sciences Center, Denver, CO 80262.   (303)-394-8251.

Rudrud, E., Rudrud, J., & Decker, D. S. *Developmental disabilities: Etiology and description*. Vermillion, S.D.: Center for the Developmentally Disabled, 1979. (Slide/tape)

Rudrud, E., Rudrud, J., & Decker, D. S. *Introduction to developmental disabilities: Historical and legal aspects*. Vermillion, S.D.: Center for the Developmentally Disabled, 1979. (Slide/tape)

REFERENCES

Aird, R. B., & Woodbury, D. M. *The management of epilepsy*. Springfield, Ill.: Charles C Thomas, 1974.

Arangio, A. J. *Behind the stigma of epilepsy*. Washington, D.C.: Epilepsy Foundation of America, 1974.

Blatt, B. *Exodus from pandemonium*. Boston: Allyn & Bacon, 1970.

Brown v. Board of Education of Topeka, Kansas, 347 U.S. 483, 493, 1954.

Donaldson v. O'Conner, 493 F. 2d 507 (5th Cir. 1974).

Finnie, H. R. *Handling the young cerebral palsied child at home*. New York: E. P. Dutton, 1974.

Gastaut, H. Clinical and electroencephalographic classification of epileptic seizures. *Epilepsia*, 1970, *11*, 102–113.

Grossman, H. J. *Manual on terminology and classification in mental retardation* (1977 revision). Washington, D.C.: American Association on Mental Deficiency, 1977.

Ingalls, R. P. *Mental retardation: The changing outlook*. New York: John Wiley & Sons, 1978.

Keats, S. *Cerebral palsy*. Springfield, Ill.: Charles C Thomas, 1965.

MacMillan, D. L. *Mental retardation in school and society*. Boston: Little, Brown, & Co., 1977.

Mills v. Board of Education of District of Columbia, United States District Court for the District of Columbia, 348 F. Supp. 866, 1972.

Pennsylvania Association for Retarded Children v. Commonwealth of Pennsylvania. 343 F. Supp. 279 (E.D., PA), 1972.

President's Committee on Mental Retardation. *MR-72: Islands of excellence.* Washington, D.C.: U.S. Government Printing Office.

Schmidt, R. P., & Wilder, B. J. *Epilepsy.* Philadelphia: F. A. Davis Co., 1968.

Souder v. Brennan, 367 F. Supp. 808 (D.C. 1973).

Thormahlen, W. A. A study of the ward training of trainable mentally retarded children in a state institution. *California Mental Health Research Monographs,* 1965, No. 5.

Ward, A. A., Jasper, H. H., & Pope, A. Clinical and experimental challenges of the epilepsies. In H. H. Jasper, A. A. Ward, & A. Pope (Eds.), *Basic mechanisms of the epilepsies.* Boston: Little, Brown, & Co., 1969.

Wolf v. Legislature of the State of Utah, Civil Action 1 82646 (3rd Jud. Dist. Ct., Utah), 1969.

Wood v. Stricklaw, Law Week, 1975, *43,* pp. 4293-4301.

Wyatt v. Stickney, 325 F. Supp. 781 (M.D. Ala. 1971).

Chapter 3

Community-Referenced Programming

OBJECTIVES

To be able to:
1. Tell why disabled persons become isolated from society.
2. Take appropriate responsibility for client goal attainment.
3. State why most developmentally disabled people come to the attention of society.
4. List those behaviors identified as critical to vocational success.
5. List the six principles of normalization.

Successful habilitation involves more than the simple application of a variety of change techniques. Which behaviors you change is as important as how you change them. This chapter is designed to provide you with information to help you choose appropriate goals for clients and to judge appropriate methodology for achieving those goals. Programs for developmentally disabled persons are increasingly moving away from large centralized institutional approaches toward community-based programs. The major reason for this is that it is believed that a program in the community ought to be better able to provide the client with those experiences necessary for integration into the mainstream of society. Thus, it is not sufficient for a community program to provide the same types of services, in the same manner, and for the same reasons as the institution. The community-based program must take advantage of the unique situations found in the community and provide community-referenced programming. That is, it must refer to the community in which it exists when setting goals.

VALUES, LABELS, AND TREATMENT CHOICES

In providing services to developmentally disabled persons, evaluation methods and treatment strategies are closely linked. That is, the way in which you view an individual and then react to that individual are nearly inseparable (Merten, 1968). As discussed in Chapter 2, there has historically been a close relationship between our basic understanding of developmental disabilities and the kinds of treatment available to developmentally disabled individuals. White and Wolfensberger (1969) described the Western concepts of mental retardation as closely linked to the philosophies of Luther and Calvin, who both perceived mentally retarded persons as being possessed by Satan. After a long period during which we paid little attention to developmentally disabled people, we entered a time when we wished to make deviant individuals not different. This period was followed by a time of concern in which individuals who were different were sheltered from society. Finally, we entered into a stage of alarm in which society was sheltered from the deviant. These last stages of concern and alarm are responsible for the development of large institutions that isolated people who were viewed as deviant. Understanding this is of critical importance for any person wishing to provide adequate programming for developmentally disabled individuals. The important lesson to be learned here is that individuals are segregated from society largely on the basis of their ability or inability to "fit in" (Goffman, 1963). In fact, 30 years ago Tredgold (1952) suggested that deficits in social skills should be the only criteria utilized in the identification of the mentally retarded.

Perceptions of the disabled not only affect federal, state, and local policy (Pollard, Hall, & Kerran, 1979), but also affect decisions made at the service delivery level. A developmentally disabled client enters a program with a vast array of useful and not so useful information, including educational history, social history, medical history, and probably scores on a variety of tests. It is likely that somewhere in the client's past, or in the immediate future, someone will provide the client with some sort of diagnostic label such as severely or profoundly retarded, cerebral palsied, or low functioning. Studies suggest that clients who are labeled in a certain way are likely to receive different types of instructor interactions (Rosenthal & Jacobson, 1968; Palmer, 1979). That is, it seems that we have let labels determine what kind of services clients will receive and what kind of goals we can expect clients to achieve.

In the past, it was assumed that people who today would be labeled as developmentally disabled could not function in society and required segregated or isolated environments. Therefore, attempts to teach them skills necessary for community integration were viewed as unnecessary. That is, their label dictated what skills were to be taught. One central assumption of this chapter is that the particular label applied to a client (whether it be the result of test scores, a categorical label, a functional label, or a formal or informal label) bears no predictive relationship to the learning potential of that client (Bellamy, O'Connor, & Karan, 1979). We believe that clients can learn, and to limit the kinds of things we expect from a person just because of a label is a great injustice. In fact, we suggest that, unless grouping and labeling somehow contribute to a change in the functional level of a client, they have very little relevance to providing programs.

Exercises
3-1. When are client "labels" useful?
3-2. What is a major problem with labels?

Answers to Exercises
3-1. When the labels lead to beneficial changes in client service delivery.
3-2. Labels often dictate how we interact with others. Think back to your first day of work. Have you had the experience of visitors who don't know whom to ask for help when they come to your center? Visitors who are unfamiliar with a program often have difficulty distinguishing staff from clients. This can result in some interesting interactions.

WHO OWNS THE PROBLEM

To truly reduce the effects of a label we must begin to change the way we evaluate clients. Rather than seeing the problem as being within the client (e.g., the client is severely retarded), we need to begin to view the problem as one of restructuring learning experiences to take advantage of the client's unique strengths and needs. When the problem is viewed as how best to individualize instruction for a particular client, we then begin to view environmental conditions as the problem.

In succeeding chapters we discuss the considerable evidence we have regarding the importance of antecedents (what comes before), task structure (what is required), and consequences (what comes after) in helping developmentally disabled persons acquire new skills. One major reason for suggesting that the problem is really in the environment is that there is not much that can be done by us about genetic abnormalities, birth defects, or biochemical malfunctions. However, antecedents, task structure, and consequences all can be directly changed and manipulated by an instructor. Thus, when the environment is the problem, the difficulty is no longer the client's failure to learn or progress but rather the instructor's problem of how best to teach the client.

This premise suggests that if the client is not learning, changing, or succeeding in a program the instructor must take responsibility. This is both good and bad news. The good news is that, through changing the environment, we can help clients change. The bad news is that *you* are responsible! However, there is a limit to this responsibility. In order to restructure learning experiences you must have a degree of control over the client's environment. If you do not have this control, there is no way you can be expected to change behavior. For example, unless you are working in or closely with a residential program, don't expect to change the client's hygiene behavior there by teaching shaving and dressing during the day program.

CAN CLIENTS LEARN PRODUCTIVE SKILLS?

We have often let our biases and expectancies control the types of programs offered to developmentally disabled clients. In the past, it was assumed that developmentally disabled individuals could not function in any kind of integrated environment. At best they could be placed in a sheltered workshop. Thus, attempts to teach these individuals the skills necessary for community and vocational integration were viewed as unnecessary. However, many authors have demonstrated that even severely mentally retarded people can master a variety of vocational skills, such as assembling a 19-piece cam switch actuator (Bellamy, Peterson, & Close, 1975) or a 79-step Tektronix cable harness (Hunter & Bellamy, 1976). Furthermore, these skills have been mastered to a level that competitive industry requires of its normal workers. Let's look at the following case study:

> In a study on severely retarded individuals' abilities to assemble the 19-piece cam switch actuator, Bellamy et al. (1975) presented data on two clients. Client 1 was a 26-year-old Down's syndrome male who had been institutionalized for 15 years. He obtained a Vineland Social Quotient of 23 and a Peabody Picture Vocabulary IQ of 10. Client 2 was a 22-year-old female institutionalized for 18 years prior to training. Her Vineland Social Quotient was 19. Both clients were taught to assemble a 19-piece cam switch actuator. Component parts ranged in size from ⅜" in length and 3/16" in diameter to 2¾" in length and 1" in diameter. The 19-piece assembly task involved 51 separate steps that were taught in a forward chain. That is, for each new step the preceding step(s) needed to be performed before the trial was reinforced. Success was defined by both clients achieving two perfect trials in a row (all 51 steps). Client 1 achieved success in 89 trials, which represented a total of 8 hours and 38 minutes of actual training. Client 2 achieved success in 6 hours and 19 minutes of training.

Similar success has been achieved in teaching independent living skills (*Detailed Progress Report,* 1970; Johnson & Bailey, 1977). The *Detailed Progress Report* (1970) from Parsons State Hospital in Kansas demonstrated success in teaching a wide variety of residential skills, including personal grooming, vocabulary building, communication skills, leisure time skills, and housekeeping skills.

SELECTING COMMUNITY-REFERENCED GOALS

Functional Behaviors

As utilized here, the term "functional behaviors" means those behaviors that 1) are needed for an individual to effectively function in potential future environments, 2) increase independent functioning, and 3) are likely to be reinforced by the environment. This means that what is taught should be determined by the demands of the present and future natural environments.

In order to successfully provide habilitation programs, behavior goals need to address functional behaviors. However, this is difficult to do. Many programs invest considerable time and effort in the development of exhaustive lists of survival skills that need to be taught to clients. The development of these skills is undeniably important, but it must be remembered that they take on a secondary importance when compared to the process, or "how" the skill is displayed. Additionally, there is no realistic way to generate an exhaustive list of all the functional behaviors that would serve in any situation. We may be able to agree on general categories (like Krantz's (1971) list of vocational behaviors—see Table 3-1), but specifics are difficult. There are just too many situational and contextual variables to consider.

By attempting to teach everything to everyone, we often dilute well-meaning efforts by keeping people in perpetual training and losing sight of the fact that there is a world that they need to enter. Even if we were to generate an exhaustive list of functional behaviors for one community, there would be little practicality in using that list in another community. Those behaviors that are functional in New York City are not necessarily needed or even appropriate on a farm in North Dakota.

A way around the problem is the view that skills become defined in terms of their critical function (Brown, Nietupski, & Hamre-Nietupski, 1976; White & Haring, 1976). There is further advantage in this approach to functional behaviors, beyond directly relating instructional objectives to *where* the student is going and *what* he or she will need on arrival. By defining the critical function, or purpose, of a skill, we can begin to identify methods of achieving that end without restricting ourselves to traditional behavior patterns.

For example, it would be redundant and uneconomical to attempt to teach a mentally retarded student to identify all of the possible names a given community can generate for men's and women's restrooms, even though knowing all of the possible names would mean increased integration within a community. However, it is possible to teach a dominant two or three names and then teach clients to ask for help when confronted with a new or novel stimulus. Thus, the critical function (appropriate use of restrooms) is achieved, but the form (i.e., complete discriminative ability) is altered. In order to define these different forms, you need to think about how many ways there are of achieving a particular goal. For example, cooking is only one method that people may utilize to achieve the goal of a balanced diet. Other ways to achieve the goal are having someone else cook the meal or eating out in restaurants and selecting a balanced diet. Bernstein (in press) suggests that we should first define the function of a behavior and then define the various methods of achieving that function.

Exercise

3-3. What are functional behaviors?

Answer to Exercise

3-3. Behaviors that:
1. Are needed for the individual to effectively function in potential future environments.
2. Will increase independent functioning.
3. Are likely to be reinforced by the environment.

Social/Emotional Skills

Although demonstrations of productive vocational and self-care potential are encouraging and important, they suffer from a major problem: they generally assume that skill development is the domain of prevocational or vocational training programs and that appropriate social and emotional behaviors, which also affect community integration, will be learned elsewhere. Overemphasis on the development of certain vocational skills or living skills can result in neglect of the most important basis for success in community integration. The simple fact is that developmentally disabled individuals come to the attention of society not because of an inability to assemble switch actuators or bicycle brakes, to perform janitorial tasks, or to tell time. Rather, developmentally disabled persons are singled out for the way they look and act. Social/emotional inappropriateness, not skill level on a particular task, is the reason most developmentally disabled people fail in community integration efforts. To maximize survival in the public sector it is critical that our clients acquire social/emotional skills in addition to specific job tasks (Rusch, 1979).

Analysis of the reasons for success or failure of developmentally disabled persons in community integration overwhelmingly points to social/emotional factors as critical elements (McCarver & Craig, 1974; Crawford, Aiello, & Thompson, 1979). Becker, Widener, and Soforenko (1979) surveyed staff of community-based vocational training programs and found social/emotional factors listed as the number one reason for job placement failure of their developmentally disabled clients. Interestingly enough, although these factors are identified as important survival skills, they are not generally emphasized in community-based programs. Mithaug and Hagmeier (1978) surveyed sheltered workshops and found that ability to communicate basic needs and move safely about the shop were identified as essential for entry into sheltered workshop programs. Social skills were rated 37th! What we know is obviously not often incorporated into our vocational training programs.

Krantz (1971) developed a list of behaviors critical for the vocational success of any person (Table 3-1). Of the 19 main categories of behavior, 17 are decidedly social/emotional in nature and only two have to do with skill level. These items were "client produces enough work" and "client produces

Table 3-1.   Critical vocational behaviors

A.   Job Objective Behaviors
  1.   Client has a vocational goal:
    a.   is oriented toward employment or having a vocational goal at all;
    b.   has a clear enough vocational goal so as to be able to move ahead at this point.

B.   Job-Getting Behaviors
  1.   Client seeks work frequently enough.
  2.   Client has appropriate interview behavior:
    a.   makes assets clear to the employer;
    b.   accounts for problems, such as periods of unemployment;
    c.   shows proper enthusiasm about the work;
    d.   is reasonably free of mannerisms which can stigmatize or annoy the employer.
  3.   Client uses job leads—knows about sources of job leads and shows this knowledge in behavior.

C.   Job-Keeping Behaviors (behaviors which help the client to stay employed after he or she gets the job)
  1.   Client attends work regularly (in general, misses less than 12 days of work per year).
  2.   Client shows up for work promptly (misses being on time no more than about 12 times per year). Note that promptness must be defined in appropriate terms; some jobs require that the employee not show up until almost exactly time to start work, and other jobs require that the person be at the work station some time before actually starting work.
  3.   Client behaves toward co-workers in such a way that:
    a.   he or she does not irritate them, make them mad, or distract them;
    b.   he or she is not abused or victimized (this would create an administrative burden to the employer).
  4.   Client behaves in relation to supervision so that:
    a.   he or she shows an acceptance of his or her subordinate role in relation to the supervisor;
    b.   he or she creates minimum supervisory overhead, consuming only ordinary supervisory time and attention.
  5.   Client produces enough work:
    a.   remains at the work station to an extent appropriate to the occupation;
    b.   maintains adequate production speed (a common problem being low productivity—rarely, a client may have too high a speed, leading to his or her rejection as a rate-buster);
    c.   sustains effort and shows adequate stamina and demonstrates willingness to continue to exert him- or herself against the demands of the work world.

(continued)

Table 3-1. (*continued*)

---

    6. Client produces up to appropriate quality standards:
        a. recognizes that there are quality standards and accepts them as reasonable demands;
        b. attends to meeting quality standards and has attained the capability of meeting them;
        c. recognizes the point of "good enough" and does not sacrifice production rate to needless perfectionism.

D. Social Living Competencies
    1. Client utilizes his or her leisure time so that he or she is:
        a. appropriately engaged and occupied rather than being at loose ends;
        b. satisfied and reasonably content with leisure time occupation.
    2. Client manages his or her money so that he or she does not spend more than income.
    3. Client has acceptable grooming and appearance.
    4. Client manages legal problems adequately (avoids excessive garnishments, manages divorce and other personal suits, and effectively manages claims against such government services as social security or unemployment compensation).

E. Community Living Competencies
    1. Client finds a place to live and maintains reasonable stability in housing.
    2. Client secures adequate medical services (rehabilitation clients, the disadvantaged, and the retarded no less than the physically disabled frequently have an unusual amount of medical needs. They frequently are plagued by a multitude of minor to serious medical problems and have shown themselves to be inept at securing services).
    3. Client is mobile in the community—uses personal or public transportation when necessary for employment, recreation, and personal affairs.

F. General and Personal Living Competencies
    1. Client copes with family and marital relationships so that they do not interfere with employment.
    2. Client has adequate personal adjustment and stability. (This is to be interpreted according to the individual and his situation and, above all, in relation to worker functioning. It is possible for a good worker to be chronically depressed or unhappy or even in acute physical pain. He or she may think odd thoughts. However, the critical behaviors are those which are emitted in such a way as to influence his or her employability.)

Adapted from: Krantz, G. Critical vocational behaviors. *Journal of Rehabilitation*, July–August, 1971.

up to appropriate quality standards." As we pointed out, even severely and profoundly retarded individuals can be taught to produce at acceptable levels. Several sources (Goldstein, 1964; Halpern, 1973) estimate that that the majority of retarded persons have the potential for satisfactory vocational and social adjustment, although this level is rarely attained (McFall, 1966; Tobias, 1970). It appears that it is not so much what developmentally disabled people do as how they go about it that is important.

Exercise

3-4. Why is it important to teach social skills?

Answer to Exercise

3-4. Because these skills can label the client. A person who acts deviant will be viewed and interacted with as being deviant.

Process Versus Product Goals

The distinction between a product, or "what," and a process, or "how," is perhaps initially confusing. It can be illustrated with the following example:

> A staff person is working on time-telling skills with a group of activity center clients utilizing a picture of a clock. The instructor asks, "Who can come to the board and point to 12 o'clock?" One client loudly proclaims that he can and, when given permission by the staff person, scrapes his chair across the floor, mutters, "I can, I can" several times on his way to the board, taps a fellow student as he passes, and walks bent over with a slow shuffle. He approaches the clock picture and correctly points to 12 o'clock. The instructor responds with "Good job, now you may sit down."

From a strictly product or "what" perspective this was indeed a good job. The client appropriately pointed to 12 o'clock. However, the process or "how" the client pointed to 12 o'clock is the real problem for this person. No matter how well time-telling skills are developed there is little hope, if any, of integration and acceptance into the community as long as his behavior, or process, remains objectionable and deviant. Thus, a primary long-term objective is to teach clients those behaviors that are necessary for acceptance in the community.

> Karen was a 22-year-old mildly retarded woman who came to the attention of one of the authors, who was then working as a consultant to a residential facility. Karen had been terminated by the local vocational rehabilitation counselor after her second behavior incident in 12 months. Her vocational placement as a motel maid had been a success with the exception of certain "incidents." Karen was considered a good worker. The problem was that periodically she would blow up and become self-abusive for "no apparent reason." Close analysis and interview of people around her indicated that Karen's incidents were closely related to criticism. A good guess about what might be causing her blowups was that her supervisor's criticism increased tension, which increased her errors, which increased the supervisor's criticism. Karen's solution to the problem was to blow up and subsequently lose her job. Although this might seem maladaptive, it was her way to escape the criticism. Through role-playing Karen was taught to respond in an appropriate verbal way to criticism from supervisors. Additionally, she was reinforced when she corrected her errors. Training, begun by role-playing, was later extended to the residential unit and finally to a number of motels in the

community. Karen was able to control her blowups and was subsequently successfully employed as a maid.

NORMALIZATION

When teaching process goals to clients, it is important to remember the principles of normalization (Nirje, 1969) and to incorporate them as part of the methodology utilized to achieve goals. We do not believe in the widespread promulgation of these principles as a sort of new religion. However, they are consistent with our belief that the environment is the location of the problem, and that the instructor must take responsibility. We view normalization principles as one more set of helpful guidelines to follow in designing habilitation programs. Thus, we normalize staff, not clients.

Wolfensberger (1972) defined normalization as the utilization of means that are as culturally normative as possible to establish and/or maintain personal behaviors and characteristics that are as culturally normative as possible. Although this may seem too simplistic, in actuality the definition is far-reaching. "As culturally normative as possible" implies that *how* behaviors are taught is as important as the behaviors to be taught. Furthermore, what is viewed as normative in one location, culture, or society may not be normal or typical in another. This statement has particular implications for age appropriateness of activities. When was the last time that you put a picture puzzle together? Yet, when a 50-year-old client is placed in an activity center, his whole day may be construction of one puzzle after another.

To establish and/or maintain personal behaviors and characteristics that are as culturally normative as possible defines the goal of habilitation training. To the fullest extent possible clients should participate in activities that society considers to be meaningful. In general, the principles of normalization refer to ensuring that clients lead a life as close to the normal as possible. Specifically, they include:

1. *A normal rhythm of the day.* If you have ever spent some time as a patient in a hospital, you know that wake-up, breakfast, lunch, and dinner occur at rather odd times. This schedule is a reflection of when shifts change in most hospitals. In applying this principle to our clients, make certain that getting up, dressing, eating, and working times are a reflection of your community's norms, not a function of staff convenience.
2. *A normal rhythm of the week.* Most of us work in one place, sleep in another, and play in still another. Clients should too! We see too many programs that utilize one or two spaces for all activities. Be creative about *where* you provide programs. Make *where* related to the norms of your community.

3. *A normal developmental life cycle.* Children, adolescents, and adults are *all* treated differently in society. Your adult clients are not children, kids, boys, or girls. They are men and women. Make certain your programs, methods, and activities reflect this!! Forty-year-olds do not usually dress up as the number one mushroom in the Christmas play. Neither should your clients. By making them seem like children you not only reinforce your (and their) thoughts and behaviors that they are children, but you perpetuate harmful community stereotypes. Correct people who refer to, program for, or behave as if all clients were children.

4. *A range of choices.* We not only insist, but expect, that this will occur at two distinct levels within your program. First, and most basic, choice for clients needs to occur at a programmatic level. That is, clients need to be involved, as much as possible, in choosing goals, methods, or programs. Even if this involvement is as little as choosing a reinforcer, it is, nonetheless, involvement. Second, we need to be aware that clients have needs and desires. If we never allow clients free choice to go or not go, stay or not stay, participate or not participate, how can we ever expect them to make appropriate choices when placed in independent situations?

5. *Living in a world of two sexes.* One reason often stated for segregation of clients (beyond the fact that it might be more convenient for staff) is that they don't know how to interact with appropriate sex partners. How in the world are clients ever going to acquire appropriate heterosocial skills if they are never given the opportunity? The world is comprised of two sexes, and client programs ought to reflect this fact!

6. *The right to economic standards.* As Bellamy, Horner, and Inman (1978) suggest, without the skills necessary to access a normal economic existence, clients will continue to receive programs that pretend to provide habilitative services via "field trips, pseudo-athletic contests, and service club sympathy parties." The technology needed to teach marketable vocational skills to even profoundly disabled individuals exists. Our programs must continually strive to apply this technology to clients. To fail to do so is to deny them access to the ways in which most people integrate into the mainstream.

Exercise
3-5. What are the six principles of normalization?

Answer to Exercise
3-5. 1. A normal rhythm of the day.
2. A normal rhythm of the week.
3. A normal developmental life cycle.
4. A range of choices.
5. Living in a world of two sexes.
6. The right to economic standards.

SUMMARY

Social competence is clearly an important aspect of providing proactive habilitation programs for clients. Stigmatizing biases have too long determined our intervention goals and strategies. These first three chapters have been intended to provide you with a philosophical framework in which to view services to developmentally disabled persons. Now that you have information about *what* to change, you are ready to read on about *how* to make change occur.

SUGGESTED ACTIVITIES

1. List labels you find in client files.
2. Use the criteria for selecting functional behaviors to evaluate client goals written in your agency.
3. Discuss with other staff how you are going to identify and teach needed social skills.
4. Determine how well your program uses the six principles of normalization. What might you change to make more use of them?

ADDITIONAL RESOURCES

Begab, M. J., & Richardson, S. A. *The mentally retarded and society: A social science perspective.* Baltimore: University Park Press, 1975.
Magrab, P. R., & Elder, J. O. *Planning for services to handicapped persons: Community, education, health.* Baltimore: Paul H. Brookes Publishing Co., 1979.

REFERENCES

Becker, R., Widener, Q., & Soforenko, A. Z. Career education for trainable mentally retarded youth. *Education and Training of the Mentally Retarded,* 1979, *14,* 101–105.
Bellamy, T., Horner, R., & Inman, D. P. *Vocational habilitation of severely retarded adults.* Baltimore: University Park Press, 1978.
Bellamy, T., O'Connor, G., & Karan, O. *Vocational rehabilitation of severely handicapped persons.* Baltimore: University Park Press, 1979.
Bellamy, T., Peterson, L., & Close, D. Habilitation of the severely and profoundly handicapped: Illustrations of competence. *Education and Training of the Mentally Retarded,* 1975, *10,* 174–186.
Bernstein, G. S. On selecting target behaviors: How many ways are there to get where we're going? *Division 25 Recorder,* in press.
Brown, L., Nietupski, J., & Hamre-Nietupski, S. *The criteria of ultimate functioning and public school services for severely handicapped students.* Madison, Wisc.: University of Wisconsin and Madison Public Schools, 1976.
Crawford, J. L., Aiello, J. R., & Thompson, D. E. Deinstitutionalization and community placement: Clinical and environmental factors. *Mental Retardation,* 1979, *17*(2), 59–63.
Detailed progress report: A demonstration program for intensive training of institutionalized mentally retarded girls (five year summary). Parsons, Kans.: Bureau

of Child Research, University of Kansas, Parsons State Hospital and Training Center, June 1965–July 1970.

Goffman, E. *Stigma: Notes on the management of spoiled identity.* Englewood Cliffs, N.J.: Prentice-Hall, 1963.

Goldstein, H. Social and occupational adjustment. In H. A. Stevens & R. Heber (Eds.), *Mental retardation: A review of research.* Chicago: University of Chicago Press, 1964.

Halpern, A. General unemployment and vocational opportunities for EMR individuals. *American Journal of Mental Deficiency,* 1973, *78,* 123–127.

Hunter, J. D., & Bellamy, T. Cable harness construction for severely retarded adults: A demonstration of training technique. In T. Bellamy (Ed.), *Habilitation of severely and profoundly retarded adults.* Eugene, Ore.: Center on Human Development, University of Oregon, 1976.

Johnson, M. S., & Bailey, J. S. The modification of leisure behavior in a half-way house for retarded women. *Journal of Applied Behavior Analysis,* 1977, *10,* 273–282.

Krantz, G. Critical vocational behaviors. *Journal of Rehabilitation,* July–August, 1971.

McCarver, R. B., & Craig, E. M. Placement of the retarded in the community: Prognosis and outcome. In N. R. Ellis (Ed.), *International review of research in mental retardation* (Vol. 7). New York: Academic Press, 1974.

McFall, T. M. Post-school adjustment: A survey of 50 former students of classes for the educable mentally retarded. *Exceptional Children,* 1966, *32,* 633–634.

Merten, R. K. The self-fulfilling prophecy. In R. K. Merten (Ed.), *Social theory and social structure.* New York: The Free Press, 1968.

Mithaug, D. E., & Hagmeier, L. D. The development of procedures to assess prevocational competencies of severely handicapped young adults. *AAESPH Review,* 1978, *3,* 94–115.

Nirje, B. The normalization principle and its human management implications. In R. B. Kugel & W. Wolfensberger (Eds.), *Changing patterns of residential care for the mentally retarded.* Washington, D.C.: PCMR, 1969.

Palmer, D. J. Regular classroom teacher's attributions and instructional prescriptions for handicapped and non-handicapped students. *Journal of Special Education,* 1979, *13,* 325–337.

Pollard, A., Hall, H., & Kerran, C. Community service planning. In P. Magrab & J. Elder (Eds.), *Planning for services to handicapped persons.* Baltimore: Paul H. Brookes Publishers, 1979.

Rosenthal, R., & Jacobson, L. *Pygmalion in the classroom.* New York: Holt, Rinehart & Winston, 1968.

Rusch, F. R. Toward the validation of social/vocational survival skills. *Mental Retardation,* 1979, *17,* 143–146.

Tobias, T. Vocational adjustment of young retarded adults. *Mental Retardation,* 1970, *8*(3), 13–16.

Tredgold, A. F. *A textbook on mental deficiency.* Baltimore: Williams and Wilkins, 1952.

White, O. R., & Haring, N. G. *Exceptional teaching: A multimedia training package.* Columbus, OH.: Charles E. Merrill Publishing Co., 1976.

White, W. D., & Wolfensberger, W. The evolution of dehumanization in our institutions. *Mental Retardation,* 1969, *7,* 5–9.

Wolfensberger, W. *The principle of normalization in human services.* Toronto: National Institute on Mental Retardation, 1972.

Unit II

Individualized Program Planning
Where Are We Going?

Chapter 4

The Planning Process

OBJECTIVES

To be able to:
1. List the six principles of Public Law (PL) 94-142.
2. List the nine essential components of an Individualized Education Program (IEP).
3. List the four purposes of assessment.
4. List seven questions that must be answered by assessment if it is to be useful in program planning.
5. List common biases of assessments.
6. List the six steps of the goal planning process.
7. List four sets of priorities that must be considered when prioritizing client goals.

PUBLIC LAW 94-142

In recent years state and federal legislation and accreditation standards have required written individualized habilitation programs for developmentally disabled individuals. The most far-reaching of these mandates were enacted by PL 94-142, the Education for All Handicapped Children Act. PL 94-142 specifically addresses children between 3 and 21 years of age. There are, however, many handicapped individuals who are over 21, and thus do not fall within the age guidelines of PL 94-142, who receive services from the Departments of Social Services and Vocational Rehabilitation and other private and public agencies. The authors believe that the principles outlined in PL 94-142 directly apply to the appropriate delivery of services to handicapped adults. In fact, many of the same principles are outlined in accreditation standards and state statutes (laws). With this in mind, an in-depth explanation of PL 94-142 is warranted.

The purpose of PL 94-142 is:

[To assure] that all handicapped children have available to them a free appropriate public education which emphasizes special education and related services designed to meet their unique needs, to assure that the rights of handicapped children and their parents or guardians are protected, to assist states and localities to provide for the education of all handicapped children, and to assess and assure the effectiveness of effort to educate handicapped children. (Sec. 601(c))

The six basic principles of PL 94-142 are: 1) zero reject, 2) nondiscriminatory testing, 3) Individualized Education Programs, 4) least restrictive environment, 5) due process, and 6) parent participation. Each of these principles are interrelated and must be considered in providing services to these individuals.

Zero Reject Principle

The principle of zero reject requires that *all* handicapped children be provided with a free, appropriate public education. These educational services are to be provided at public expense, must meet the standards of the state educational agency, must be in conformity with the Individualized Education Program, and must include preschool, elementary, or secondary educational services. As of September 1, 1980, states were required to provide these educational services to all handicapped children 3 to 21 years of age.

Nondiscriminatory Evaluation Principle

The principle of nondiscriminatory evaluation requires that a handicapped student must receive a complete individual evaluation prior to placement in a special education program. The evaluation is the first step in providing appropriate educational services. The evaluation procedures must meet the following standards (*Federal Register*, 1977, pp. 42496–42497):

1. Tests and other evaluation materials:
   a. are provided and administered in the child's native language or other mode of communication, unless it is clearly not feasible to do so;
   b. have been validated for the specific purpose for which they are used; and
   c. are administered by trained personnel in conformance with the instructions provided by their producer.
2. Tests and other evaluation materials include those tailored to assess specific areas of educational need and not merely those which are designed to provide a single general intelligence quotient.
3. Tests are selected and administered so as best to ensure that when a test is administered to a child with impaired sensory, manual, or speaking skills, the test results accurately reflect the child's aptitude or achievement level rather than reflecting the child's impaired sensory, manual, or

speaking skills (except where those skills are the factors which the test purports to measure). For example, tests that require timed motor tasks are not appropriate tests for individuals with motor impairments unless you are specifically addressing those motor skills.

4. No single procedure is used as the sole criterion for determining an appropriate educational program for a child.
5. The evaluation is made by a multidisciplinary team or group of persons, including at least one teacher or other specialist with knowledge in the area of suspected disability.
6. The child is assessed in all areas related to the suspected disability, including, where appropriate, health, vision, hearing, social and emotional status, general intelligence, academic performance, communicative status, and motor abilities.

Individualized Education Program

After the evaluation has been completed and the student has been identified as needing special education services, the next step is the development of an Individualized Education Program (IEP). As stipulated in PL 94-142, an IEP must be written for every handicapped student who is receiving special education or related services. Each IEP must include the following:

1. Documentation of the student's present level of educational performance, including academic achievement, social adaptation, prevocational and vocational skills, physical education, and self-help skills.
2. Annual goals that describe the educational performance to be achieved by the end of the school year.
3. Short-term instructional objectives that are the measurable intermediate steps between the present level of educational performance and the annual goals.
4. Documentation of the specific special education and related services needed by the child. These are to be determined without regard to the availability or cost of those services.
5. Justification for the type of educational placement that the student will have and an indication of the extent of time the student will participate in regular education programs.
6. Projected dates for when those services will begin and the length of time the services will be given.
7. Identification of individuals who are responsible for the implementation of the Individualized Education Program.
8. Objective criteria, evaluation procedures, and schedules for determining mastery of short-term objectives at least on an annual basis.
9. Documentation regarding the extent to which the child will participate in regular education programs.

Basically, handicapped students who require adaptation of the regular curriculum, regardless of placement, must have an IEP developed for those aspects of the curriculum that are adapted. Some students will require an IEP for every academic subject and other students may require an IEP for one particular area of deficit. For example, a learning disabled student who has difficulties in arithmetic but not in other subjects may require an IEP in arithmetic but not in science, history, physical education, and so on. Furthermore, the IEP should not be restricted only to academic subject areas. In PL 94-142, areas to be given consideration include academic achievement, social adaptation/adjustment, prevocational and vocational skills, psychomotor skills, physical education, and self-help skills.

Each public agency is responsible for conducting meetings to develop, review, and revise a handicapped student's IEP. Each handicapped student's IEP is to be implemented at the beginning of the school year and must be reviewed at least once a year.

Each handicapped student has an IEP committee. The IEP committee should reflect the interdisciplinary process and is charged with overseeing all steps of the IEP process, including assessment, development, implementation, and review (see Figure 4-1). The IEP committee should be comprised of the following:

1. A person other than the student's teacher who has the responsibility for providing or supervising the special education services.
2. The student's teacher (special and/or regular).
3. The parents or guardians of the student.
4. The student.
5. Other individuals and/or advocates at the request of the parents or public agency.
6. Specialists who have conducted the student's evaluation or a person who is knowledgeable about the evaluation procedures used and the interpretation of the evaluation results.

Parental participation is essential to the development of the IEP. PL 94-142 states that public agencies are required to encourage parent and/or guardian participation at IEP meetings by:

1. Notifying the parents and/or guardians of the purpose, time, and location of the meeting early enough so that they have an opportunity to attend.
2. Scheduling the meeting at a mutually agreed time and location.
3. Ensuring that the parent(s) understand the proceedings of the meeting. This includes providing an interpreter for parents and/or guardians who are deaf or whose language is other than English.
4. Providing a copy of the student's IEP to the parents and/or guardians.

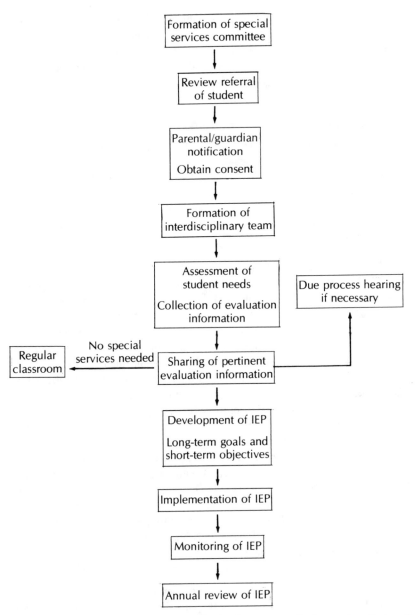

Figure 4-1. Flowchart of IEP process, used for development, coordination, and monitoring of the IEP.

If the parents and/or guardians cannot attend the scheduled IEP meetings they may participate through individual or conference telephone calls. IEP meetings may occur without parental and/or guardian input only when the parents and/or guardians have rejected all attempts by the public agency to have them involved. The agency must provide documentation of the efforts to include the parents and/or guardians.

Least Restrictive Environment Principle

The fourth principle of PL 94-142 is the placement of students in the least restrictive environment. This means that to the fullest extent possible handicapped students should receive educational programs with students who are not handicapped. Provision of educational services in special classes and/or separate facilities should occur only when handicapping conditions prevent students from participating in a regular classroom with the use of supplementary aids and services.

Due Process

The principle of due process refers to procedures that assure the appropriateness of the educational decisions and the accountability of those individuals (IEP team) who make the decisions. A due process hearing may be initiated by the parents or public agency in order to present complaints regarding a student's identification as handicapped, evaluation, placement, IEP development, or IEP implementation or to challenge decisions made by the IEP team or other individuals. The due process hearing must be conducted by the public agency that is directly responsible for the student's education. The hearing officer must have no personal or professional interest that would conflict with his or her objectivity. For instance, the hearing officer may not be an employee of the public agency.

If either the parents or the public agency are dissatisfied with the findings of the initial due process hearing they may appeal to the state education agency. The state education agency then has the responsibility for conducting an impartial review of the hearing and making an independent decision based on the review process. The decisions reached by the state education agency are considered final unless a civil action is brought against the state education agency in either a state or federal district court.

Other due process safeguards outlined in PL 94-142 include:

1. The parents and/or guardians may obtain an independent educational evaluation, at public expense, if they are dissatisfied with the evaluation obtained by the public agency.
2. The parents and/or guardians must be provided with written notification prior to evaluating or determining the student's educational placement. The notification must include:

    a. A listing of the due process safeguards available to the parent and/or guardian.

    b. A justification and description of the action taken by the public agency.

    c. A description of the process by which the decision was reached (i.e., evaluation procedures, tests, records, and reports used.)

    d. The use of language that is understood by the general public and/or a native language that the parent understands.

3. Parental and/or guardian consent must be obtained prior to conducting the evaluation to determine if the student needs special education services.

4. If the public agency is unable to contact the student's parents, the agency must assign an individual to act as a surrogate for the parents. This individual is charged with the responsibility to represent the child in all matters regarding the provision of free and appropriate educational services.

Parental Participation

The final principle of PL 94-142 regards parental participation. Parents and/or guardians have the right to be involved in the IEP process. Furthermore, the parents and/or guardians may review any educational records that are used by the agency before or after meeting to develop the student's IEP.

Parental and guardian participation extends beyond the IEP process. Parents and/or guardians are to be involved in the development and approval of educational policy. The state education agency is responsible for developing a state education plan that specifies how the educational needs of handicapped students will be met. As stated in PL 94-142, parents and/or guardians are encouraged to participate in public hearings and to become members of advisory boards and panels in efforts to shape the state plan for the education of handicapped students. Additionally, the local education agencies are required to provide the opportunity for the parents and/or guardians of handicapped students to express their views and opinions as to how PL 94-142 funds are allocated.

In summary, PL 94-142 assures that all handicapped children (ages 3 to 21) will have a free appropriate public education that is designed to meet their unique needs. All state and local education agencies must comply with all of the requirements of PL 94-142. There are no universal IEP forms or documents, and each agency may develop its own. However, these forms must meet all of the essential requirements of the law.

Exercises

4-1. List and describe the six basic principles of PL 94-142.

4-2. List the nine essential components of an IEP.

Answers to Exercises

4-1. *Zero reject*—The principle of zero reject requires that *all* handicapped children be provided with a free appropriate public education.
Nondiscriminatory evaluation—This principle refers to the use of unbiased or culture-free assessment instruments.
Individualized Education Programs—Each handicapped child must have a written IEP.
Least restrictive environment—This principle states that to the fullest extent possible handicapped students should receive educational programs with students who are not handicapped. Placement in a regular classroom is preferred over placement in a special classroom and placement in a special classroom is preferred over placement in an institutional setting.
Due process—The principle of due process refers to procedures that assure the appropriateness of educational decisions.
Parental participation—The final principle states that parents and/or guardians have the right to be involved in the IEP process.

4-2. 1. Documentation of the student's present level of performance.
2. Annual goals.
3. Short-term instructional objectives.
4. Documentation of services needed.
5. Justification for the type of educational placement.
6. Beginning dates and lengths of time of services.
7. Identification of individuals responsible for the IEP implementation.
8. Objective criteria, evaluation procedures, and schedules for determining mastery of short-term objectives at least on an annual basis.
9. Documentation regarding the extent to which the child will participate in regular education programs.

INTERDISCIPLINARY TEAMS

PL 94-142 requires the formation of an interdisciplinary team. The interdisciplinary team is the key to the provision of successful services. The responsibilities of the interdisciplinary team are to collect, interpret, and report information for evaluation and program planning (Turnbull, Strickland, & Brantley, 1978). The size and composition of the interdisciplinary team will vary according to the severity and complexity of the client's problems. PL 94-142 specifies that the interdisciplinary team must be composed of at least one professional with expertise in the area of suspected disability. The majority of handicapped individuals receiving special services require the input of more than one professional.

The basic responsibilities of the interdisciplinary team are to collect, interpret, and report information necessary for appropriate program planning. When providing services to handicapped individuals, the majority of time the handicapped individual will be receiving services from a variety of professions. It is not uncommon to have a client who is receiving medical, psychological, physical therapy, occupational therapy, speech, rehabilitation, and special education services on a daily or weekly basis. As you can see, the

Table 4-1. Composition of an interdisciplinary team

Must be involved	May be involved	
	Agencies	Professionals
Client	Public or private special	Physicians
Parent or guardian	service agencies	Psychologists
Teacher/instructor	Visually impaired	Nurses
Agency providing services	School for the deaf	Social workers
Direct care staff	Rehabilitation	Rehabilitation counselors
Case managers	Special education	Physical therapists
	Vocational education	Adaptive physical educators
	Public health	Speech/language therapists
	Social services	Psychiatrists
	Secondary education	Special educators
	State institutions	

size of the interdisciplinary team can be immense. Table 4-1 shows a list of potential members of an interdisciplinary team.

The underlying philosophy of the interdisciplinary team is that we all come from different backgrounds, with different training and different experiences. Therefore, we may not always perceive the same problem in the same way. When the basic problem presented to the interdisciplinary team is to provide the most appropriate programming for a client, the best plan will come from a melding of perceptions of the individual team members. Unfortunately, interdisciplinary teams often lose sight of the original objective of developing the most appropriate program for the client and become battle-grounds over who is right and who is wrong or forums for professional pontification. (Effective team functioning is discussed in Chapters 14, 15, and 16 of this text.) Nevertheless, it is important to remember that there is no one individual who has the expertise, knowledge, or skill to collect, interpret, and report the pertinent information from all of the agencies and professions who provide services to a particular client. This is best accomplished through an interdisciplinary team that allows all professionals to share their thoughts and findings in order to provide a more complete and coordinated approach to client programming.

ASSESSMENT

In providing services to handicapped individuals it is necessary to know where you are before you begin the habilitation program. In other words, it is necessary to conduct an assessment of the client's abilities and needs prior to providing remedial programming. Assessment can serve four purposes: diagnosis, placement, prediction, and prescription.

Diagnosis refers to conducting an assessment to determine the "cause" of the problem. For example, if we went to our family physician complaining of a fever and small spots on our skin, an assessment might lead to a diagnosis of a case of measles. The assessment procedures have resulted in a diagnosis, but the diagnosis in and of itself does not remedy our situation. Similarly, a diagnosis of "mental retardation," "cerebral palsy," "minimal brain dysfunction," or "epilepsy" are outcomes of assessment procedures, but the client is no better and sometimes worse off once he or she is diagnosed. Oftentimes, diagnosis will lead to labeling that is detrimental to the client (see Chapter 3 for a discussion of this issue).

Another outcome of assessment may be *placement*. Placement refers to an outcome in which individuals who "score" similarly on an assessment battery receive special services that are designed to serve special groups. Twenty years ago, to be diagnosed as mentally retarded most likely meant that you would be placed in a state institution. Assessment-related placements continue today. There are now special programs for students who are diagnosed as being visually impaired, hearing impaired, culturally disadvantaged, educable mentally retarded, or severely/profoundly mentally retarded. Thus, assessment can lead to placement rather than remediation.

Assessment procedures may also result in *prediction*. Prediction refers to determining an outcome prior to its occurrence based upon assessment information. Intelligence tests were designed to be predictive. One of the first intelligence tests was developed by French psychologists Binet and Simon. They were commissioned by the Minister of Public Education to develop a test that would identify children who were too dull to benefit from regular schooling (Ingalls, 1978). In other words, a child's performance on the intelligence test would predict whether he or she would benefit from regular school. Intelligence tests today continue to have predictive value in identifying students who will have difficulty in regular classrooms. For example, a student with an IQ score of 70 will likely have a more difficult time in a regular classroom than a student with an IQ score of 115.

Although prediction can identify outcomes, prediction does not lead to remediation of problems. The most important purpose of assessment is *prescription*. Prescription refers to what can be done to remediate the problem. Knowing that a handicapped individual is diagnosed as having Down's syndrome, has an IQ score of 63, and is currently enrolled in a self-contained special education classroom does not provide useful information for programming.

When conducting an assessment for the purpose of prescription it is useful to ask the following questions:

1. What can the individual do? What are the individual's strengths?
2. What type and how much assistance do you have to supply? Under what conditions?
3. What are the individual's needs?
4. What resources does your agency have that can meet the individual's needs?
5. What teaching techniques have been successful with the individual?
6. What teaching techniques have been unsuccessful?
7. What positive and negative experiences has the individual had that may influence programming?

These questions provide a framework for prescription, that is, for developing appropriate program planning that will set realistic expectations and goals.

Limitations of Assessment Information

PL 94-142 requires that sources of bias in the process of identifying and classifying handicapped students must be eliminated. In other words, the assessment tool used to assess the student's abilities must not penalize the student because of the nature of the assessment process. Sources of bias are numerous and may include the following:

Cultural Background   In a society that is as diverse as ours many differences exist within each "subculture." The environment of a lower-class child has been described as being less verbally and visually stimulating and more noisy than the environment of a middle- or upper-class child, which can affect scores on tests of auditory discrimination, attention, and memory. There are many other types of cultural limitations. One question on a standardized achievement test is "What are the seasons of the year?" Most of us would respond with winter, spring, summer, and fall. However, if you live on the island of Bermuda it is common knowledge that there are only three seasons: "wet," "dry," and "hurricane." Another common response made by children who live in the western states is that the seasons of the year are deer, duck, trout, and pheasant (referring to the hunting and fishing seasons). The point is that individuals from different cultures may respond differently to a standard assessment question. As a result, some individuals are penalized unfairly by certain assessment procedures.

Native Language   Most standardized assessment tests (intelligence, achievement, abilities) are administered in the English language. This presents a problem when the handicapped individual does not speak English or when English is not the dominant language spoken in the home. In order to minimize this source of bias, a test standardized for administration and scoring in a non-English language or a nonverbal assessment instrument should be administered. If this is not possible, another alternative would be to translate the test into the individual's dominant language. During the mid 1970s many Cambodian refugees came to the United States. This presented a major obstacle to many school districts who had to place these children in appropriate educational settings. Since many of the children did not speak English, their performance on standardized tests would have placed them in special education classrooms—one cannot give the right answer when one does not understand the question.

Subjective Information   Another major source of bias is the reliance of team members on subjective opinions and information. Subjective information is based on the team members' opinions rather than on recorded data or other standardized test results. Since team members have different educational backgrounds, training experiences, and expertise, each team member will perceive and interpret client problems differently. Without accurately recorded data to document the problem no agreement as to what the problem is can occur. For example, at one client's staff meeting the special education teacher reported that the client was not attending to work and engaged in many off-task behaviors. The nurse suggested the possibility of a medical evaluation to determine if medication would be helpful. The parents reported no difficulty in having their daughter work at home and suggested their daughter did not like the special education teacher. The vocational training coordinator reported that the client was a competent worker and that she enjoyed working in the shop. In fact, it was difficult to get her to leave the shop to go to special education classes. Each team member was reporting the problem as he/she perceived it and each member perceived it differently.

It is foolhardy to attempt to solve such a problem without first obtaining data that accurately reflect the problem. A problem cannot be solved until it is defined. Relying on subjective reports for program development often results in the misallocation of resources and the development of programs that will end in failure. To overcome this bias one needs to objectively record data using one of the procedures described in Chapter 6.

Other Sources   Other sources of bias include the individual's health, nutrition, physical, visual, hearing, and speech abilities. Each of these sources must be considered when performing an assessment evaluation. An individual who has been described as lacking motivation or interest or who is lackluster and listless may be exhibiting signs of malnutrition, health problems, and so on. An appropriate assessment should address each of these areas of bias and attempt to minimize their impact on the evaluation.

How to Minimize Bias

After sources of bias have been identified the appropriateness of assessment devices must be determined. Most often this involves determining if an assessment tool has been validated for use with cultural minorities, foreign languages, communication deficits, and other handicapping conditions. There are few standardized tests available for specific cultural groups or for individuals who speak a foreign language. As a result, conclusions reached during the evaluation may be incorrect because an assessment tool was incorrectly applied.

Norm-referenced tests are designed to compare one person's performance to that of other individuals with similar characteristics. Norm-referenced tests are standardized on groups of individuals of certain ages and economic/cultural/educational backgrounds. The range of economic/cultural/educational groups included in the standardization of the test determines the populations for which the test is designed. The following characteristics are usually considered when standardizing a test: sex, age/grade, ethnic group, socioeconomic status, geographic region, urban/rural residence, setting, and on occasion handicapping conditions and IQ level. Many intelligence, achievement, and adaptive behavior assessment devices are not normed or standardized on developmentally disabled individuals or individuals with other handicapping conditions. Thus, they may be incorrectly applied. Turnbull, Strickland, and Brantley (1978) listed the following limitations of common tests (pp. 83–85):

Test	Consideration/Limitation
Slosson Intelligence Test	Questionable norms, reliability, and validity.
Stanford-Binet	Questionable norms.
Peabody Individual Achievement Test	Questionable reliability and validity. Inadequate for classification or program planning decisions.
Wide Range Achievement Test	Inadequate norms and validity. Questionable reliability. Inadequate for screening, classification, or program planning.
AAMD Adaptive Behavior Scale—Public School Version	Inadequate rules for interpreting scores, reliability, and validity. Inadequate for classification, questionable for program planning.
Vineland Social Maturity Scale	Inadequate norms, reliability, and validity. Inadequate for classification, questionable for program planning.

Exercises

4-3. Describe the major functions of the interdisciplinary team.
4-4. List and describe the four purposes of assessment.
4-5. What questions need to be addressed during assessment?
4-6. What are common biases that may occur during the evaluation process?

Answers to Exercises

4-3. The responsibilities of the interdisciplinary team are to collect, interpret, and report information for evaluation and program planning.

4-4. 1. Diagnosis refers to conducting an assessment to determine the "cause" of the problem.
    2. Placement refers to providing special services to individuals with similar needs.
    3. Prediction refers to determining an outcome prior to its occurrence based upon assessment information.
    4. Prescription refers to what can be done to remediate the problem.

4-5. 1. What can the individual do? What are the individual's strengths?
    2. What type and how much assistance to you have to supply? Under what conditions?
    3. What are the individual's needs?
    4. What resources does your agency have that can remediate the individual's needs?
    5. What teaching techniques have been successful with the individual?
    6. What teaching techniques have been unsuccessful?
    7. What positive and negative experiences has the individual had that may influence programming?

4-6. Biases may include cultural background, native language other than English, physical, speech, or health disabilities, and the use of subjective information.

THE INDIVIDUALIZED PLANNING PROCESS

There are many names associated with individual plans—for example, Individualized Education Program (IEP), or Individualized Habilitation Program (IHP). The term IPP (Individualized Program Plan) is used here to describe individualized plans.

The individualized planning process is the most important procedure in providing services to handicapped individuals. This process establishes goals to be worked on during a 12-month period and is a "contract" between the agency and the client for what services are to be provided and what expectaions are placed on the staff and client. The plans must be developed jointly by the individuals/programs who are providing services and the individual who is receiving services and, where appropriate, that individual's parents and/or guardians. The plans must include long-term (annual) goals and short-term objectives. The objectives are to be in sequence and written in behavioral terms that provide a measure of the client's progress. The plan should contain a statement of what specific educational and habilitation services are to be provided, who shall provide the services, when the services shall start, how the goals and objectives are to be achieved, the evaluation procedures, and the schedule for determining whether the objectives and goals are being achieved. The steps required in the individualized planning process are:

1. Involve the client.
2. List client strengths.
3. List client needs.

4. List and prioritize client goals.
5. List strategies to accomplish the goals.
6. Develop the Individualized Program Plan.

Involve the Client

It is difficult to imagine a meeting that will determine what you are going to be doing 24 hours a day during the next year taking place without you, but this happens when the client is not involved in the individualized planning process. The planning team is responsible for setting annual goals, and it is essential for the client to be involved to the fullest extent possible. For the client who can express his or her desires, inclusion in the planning process can help gain commitment to goal achievement, temper unrealistic client expectations, and individualize IPP methodology. Though we expect you always to individualize IPP methodology, in our experience the client's presence forces planning teams to address the client as a person, not simply as a case, a number, or a thing.

For clients whose ability to express themselves is limited, "involvement to the fullest extent possible" may mean indicating a preference among reinforcers or pointing to pictures of tasks to learn next. In any event, the client's presence serves to remind the team that the client is a person, not an abstract idea.

In general, the client should be involved in the IPP process from the beginning. Treat the client the way that you would like to be treated. In other words, ask questions and explain rather than lecture or dictate. Always explain the long-term goals and short-term objectives to the client.

List Client Strengths

It is advantageous to use client strengths when working on goals to meet client needs. Strengths are those skills and abilities the client can do or likes to do. Regardless of what some team members may say, all clients have strengths. Many new approaches to the client's needs can be identified by providing a list of abilities and skills. One client, for example, was to learn a shape discrimination task. Several approaches had been tried unsuccessfully in the past. By making a list of the client's strengths it was found that the client had mastered color discrimination. By coloring each shape differently and then fading the colors, teaching shape discrimination became a simple task (see Chapter 9 for further explanation of the fading procedure). Another client was able to change the saw blades on a table and radial arm saw. This client needed to increase his socialization with other clients. Several other clients' needs included learning to change the blades on the table and radial arm saws. By pairing his strengths with others' needs, the client who needed to increase his socialization with other clients accomplished this by teaching those clients who needed to learn how to change saw blades.

List Client Needs

Needs refer to those skills and abilities the client has not mastered, as well as to problems that affect program success (e.g., medical, financial). By writing the list of needs, it is possible to see if overlap exists between several needs that may then be combined into one need. The IPP process should involve careful analysis of need statements in order to ensure that stated needs accurately represent actual needs. For example, a case manager began a team meeting by suggesting that the client's real need was to stop telling obscene jokes and making lewd comments. Most team members initially agreed. However, a review of the strengths and needs list showed that some staff felt the client's main strength was a good sense of humor. The team then realized that the actual problem was in their differing perceptions of what was humorous.

When making the list of client needs, we strongly suggest that the needs be stated positively in terms of what the client *should* be doing rather than what he *should not* be doing. For example, "Jim needs to increase the amount of time spent at his work station" rather than "Jim needs to decrease the number of times he leaves his work station." This is done because programs designed to increase behaviors rely on positive reinforcement techniques (programs designed to decrease behaviors utilize other techniques). Positive reinforcement is the best technique available to teach new behaviors. Stating the client's needs positively makes it necessary to utilize proactive techniques.

When making the list of client strengths and needs, it is best to be as specific as possible. However, general statements may be utilized initially. These statements will become more specific when goals are identified. For example, Sally may need to increase her grooming and personal hygiene skills. This need may later be refined to a specific skill, such as "Sally will shower every morning."

The list of client needs should be determined without regard to the cost of services or to the availability of such services. For example, if the team feels that the client needs a physical therapy assessment, then that should be addressed even if the agency does not have a physical therapist. Turnbull, Strickland, and Brantley (1978) report that many educational problems of handicapped students can be attributed to failing to provide instructions based on their particular profile of strengths and weaknesses.

Prioritizing Client Goals

It is necessary for the IPP team to prioritize the client's needs into those goals that are to be worked on during the next year. The agency providing services has a limited amount of resources—that is, of time, people, equipment, educational materials, etc. As a result, it is critical to allocate those resources to meet the needs of the clients. Since it is usually impossible to meet all of the client's needs, it is necessary to choose specific goals that will be worked on during the next year. There are many ways to prioritize goals. The list below represents the authors' viewpoints.

1. *Client priorities.* This is the most important factor in prioritization. What are the client's goals? Which areas does the client want to work on? Does the client engage in behaviors that are dangerous? If so, these should be worked on immediately and oftentimes require a high allocation of available resources.
2. *Parental/guardian priorities.* What vocational/habilitation skills do the parents want to see accomplished? Oftentimes clarification of agency goals and parental expectations must occur (see below).
3. *Community priorities.* Community priorities include what services and jobs are available for training and how the community defines "normal." Training a client to strip furniture as a vocation does not do any good if there are no job opportunities in the community for furniture strippers.
4. *Agency priorities.* What types of clients does the agency serve and what services does the agency provide? When a client is referred for services, you may find his or her needs can best be met at another agency. To provide services to such a client is in reality doing a disservice.

Problems in goal planning result when there is conflict among client, parental/guardian, community, and agency priorities. The client may have unrealistic expectations and may not understand what shop skills have to do with being a surgeon. Similarly, parents may want to place their 35-year-old "child" in a "safe" program where their "child" will be cared for the rest of his or her life. Communities may resent having "retards" living in their neighborhoods and residential programs may suffer. Finally, an agency may not want to place its more productive clients in competitive jobs because the agency's production of pallets will drop.

These are just a sample of the problems in prioritizing client goals. To avoid these problems it is necessary to come back to the basic reason habilitation programs are designed: to provide habilitation training for the client so that the client may live as independently as possible. It is necessary to review all priorities and resolve conflicting expectations.

List Strategies

After the goals have been prioritized and agreed upon it is helpful to develop a list of strategies that will explain how each goal will be accomplished. As stated earlier, each team member comes from a different background with different experiences. It is not uncommon to develop a list of four or five strategies designed to teach a particular behavior. The team members should weigh the merits of each approach and make the decision as to which one to implement. Additionally, if the selected strategy does not work, alternative strategies will have already been suggested.

Individualized Program Plan

The final step in the IPP process is to develop the Individualized Program Plan. It is the team's responsibility to identify which goals will be worked on, write long-term goals and short-term objectives, and develop an evaluation plan. These topics are discussed in the next chapter.

SUMMARY

The Individualized Program Plan process results in an agreement between consumers and providers as to what services are to be provided and what expectations there are for the client. The exact IPP process varies with state, local, and facility guidelines. However, the basic principles as described in this chapter provide guidelines for effective client planning. It is essential to involve the client in the IPP process since he or she is the one who is most affected by it.

Exercises

4-7. List and describe the six steps of the goal planning process.
4-8. List and discuss four sets of priorities that must be considered when prioritizing client goals.

Answers to Exercises

4-7. 1. Involve the client.
2. List client strengths.
3. List client needs.
4. List and prioritize client goals.
5. List strategies to accomplish the goals.
6. Develop the Individualized Program Plan.
4-8. 1. Client priorities.
2. Parental/guardian priorities.
3. Community priorities.
4. Agency priorities.

SUGGESTED ACTIVITIES

1. PL 94-142 specifies six principles that directly relate to habilitation programming. These are zero reject, nondiscriminatory testing, Individualized Education Pro-

grams, least restrictive environment, due process, an/
tion. How does your agency assure that these princi

2. Obtain a copy of *The Eighth Mental Measurements*
   versity libraries have copies of this in the reference section,.
   the critiques of tests that have been administered during client ev⌐
   positive features and drawbacks of the tests administered.
3. There are nine essential components of an IPP. Review your facility's IPP form
   and evaluate whether or not it addresses each component.
4. Follow one of your clients through the IEP flowchart (Figure 4-1).
5. Compare the composition of your interdisciplinary team with that in Table 4-1.
6. How do you resolve conflicts in priorities?

ADDITIONAL RESOURCES

Barton, E. Assessing the employability of the trainable mentally retarded—tools and issues. *Vocational Evaluation and Work Adjustment Bulletin,* 1975, *8*(2), 42–58.

Bolton, B. *Handbook of measurement and evaluation in rehabilitation.* Baltimore: University Park Press, 1976.

Buros, O. K. *The eighth mental measurements yearbook.* Highland Park, N.J.: Gryphon, 1978.

Cone, J. D., & Hawkins, R. P. (Eds.) *New directions in clinical psychology.* New York: Brunner/Mazel, 1977.

Gellman, W. Principles of vocational evaluation. *Rehabilitation Literature,* 1968, *29*(4), 98–102.

Hardy, R. E., & Cull, J. G. *Vocational evaluation for rehabilitation services.* Springfield, Ill.: Charles C Thomas, 1973.

Luce, D., & Mueller, L. Evaluating the severely disabled, a case study. *Rehabilitation Review,* 1975, *1*(1).

Poor, C. Vocational potential assessment. *Archives of Physical Medicine and Rehabilitation,* 1975, *56,* 33–36.

Popovich, D. *A prescriptive behavioral checklist for the severely and profoundly retarded.* Baltimore: University Park Press, 1977.

Rehabilitation manual. Washington, D.C.: Goodwill Industries of America, 1974.

Sulzer-Azaroff, B., & Mayer, D. R. *Applying behavior analysis procedures with children and youth.* New York: Holt, Rinehart & Winston, 1977.

Tests and measurements for vocational evaluators. Menomonie, Wisc.: Materials Development Center, University of Wisconsin–Stout, 1973.

REFERENCES

Ingalls, R. P. *Mental retardation: The changing outlook.* New York: John Wiley & Sons, 1978.

Turnbull, A. P., Strickland, B. B., & Brantley, J. C. *Developing and implementing individualized education programs.* Columbus, Oh.: Charles E. Merrill, 1978.

Chapter 5

Writing Plans and Objectives

OBJECTIVES

To be able to:
1. List four components of a long-term objective.
2. List five components that may be included in a short-term objective.
3. List components of a program methodology.
4. Write a long-term objective that contains the four necessary components.
5. Write a short-term objective that contains the necessary components.

WHY DO WE WRITE IPPs?

Individualized Program Plans (IPPs) are mandated by state and federal legislation and accreditation standards; however, this should not be considered as the only reason for developing and implementing IPPs. Individualized Program Plans improve training and service delivery through:

1. Coordination of planning and programming.
2. Development of a sequential plan.
3. Specification of individual needs and services.
4. Systematic evaluation.
5. Increased professional accountability.
6. Improved communication with consumers.

Coordination of Planning and Programming

Individualized Program Plans are developed by a team. As the individualized plan is developed the team members can coordinate their efforts to meet the individualized needs of their handicapped clients and to ensure effective implementation of these plans. Coordination of programming will be enhanced by specifying the responsibilities of each team member. Furthermore, such specification will decrease the chance that an objective is not accomplished because team members assumed other team members were responsible for the completion of that objective.

Most importantly, the IPP process allows for coordination of the handicapped student's program between the agency providing services and the home. As the parents and/or guardians participate in the IPP process, they become more knowledgeable about the services being provided, and have the opportunity to provide these services at home. Greater gains can be expected when there is consistency of service being provided at the agency and at home. Coordination and consistency can eliminate the often reported setbacks after home visits, when specific programs were not followed by the parents and/or guardians. For example, an agency may be teaching handicapped individuals to dress themselves, but the effectiveness of this instruction may be lessened if their parents continue to dress them when they are at home.

Development of a Sequential Plan

Turnbull, Strickland, and Brantley (1978) reported that teachers often commented that they did not know what they would be teaching next month, much less what skills they would be teaching next semester or by the end of the school year. Furthermore, teachers were uncertain as to which skills and concepts were appropriate to their students' needs. The result of this uncertainty has often been a disjointed and random approach, similar to Alice's journey in *Alice's Adventures in Wonderland* by Lewis Carroll. During Alice's journey through Wonderland, she came to a fork in the road. She stopped, puzzled as to which direction she should take. She spied the Cheshire Pussy Cat.

> "Cheshire Puss," she began rather timidly as she did not at all know if it would like the name: However it only grinned a little wider.... "Would you tell me please which way I ought to walk from here?"
> "That depends a good deal on where you want to get to," said the Cat.
> "I don't much care where—" said Alice.
> "Then it doesn't matter which way you walk," said the Cat.
> "—so long as I get somewhere! Alice added as an explanation.
> "Oh you're sure to do that," said the Cat. "If only you walk long enough."
> (pp. 89–90)

You must know where you are going if you want to get there.

The Individualized Program Plan requires the specification of annual goals and short-term objectives. Short-term objectives are intermediate steps between the individual's present level of functioning and the accomplishment of the annual goals. As a result, the short-term objectives are sequential and relate to increasing levels of complexity and mastery. In other words, the

Individualized Program Plan must reflect a step-by-step development of skills and abilities.

The individualized planning process presents an opportunity for service providers, the handicapped individual, and parents and/or guardians to systematically plan services. When annual goals and short-term objectives are specified in advance, the handicapped individual can make increased progress and instructional time can be more effectively and efficiently used.

Specification of Individual Needs and Services

The individualized planning process focuses attention on the unique needs of a handicapped individual. Team members must consider evaluation results, current level of functioning in educational, vocational, and independent living areas, the strengths and needs of the individual, and areas of concern expressed by the individual as well as those expressed by the parents and/or guardians. The needs of the handicapped person should be determined without regard to cost or availability of services. In other words, the focal point of the planning process is the unique needs of the client rather than external factors.

We are aware, of course, that the resources needed may not exist within your agency or community. Regardless of the availability of these services, the client's total needs must be addressed in the IPP. Failure to document the need for resources decreases the possibility that these services will become available in the future.

Systematic Evaluation

The development of an Individualized Program Plan requires evaluations at three times: prior to, during, and after the IPP implementation. As mentioned in Chapter 4, prior to the development of the IPP, a handicapped individual must receive an appropriate nondiscriminatory evaluation to determine: 1) whether or not the individual is handicapped, 2) strengths and needs of the individual, 3) if special or related services are required, 4) the individual's current level of performance, and 5) appropriate goals for the individual.

During implementation of the IPP, evaluation occurs as an outgrowth of the specification of short-term objectives. The specification of short-term objectives provides a means of ongoing evaluation in terms of how the client is progressing in accomplishing the objectives and how well the specific program is working. Suppose a short-term goal for a client was that he or she was to master 12 steps of a program and upon review it was noted that the client had only accomplished two steps. Questions that may be raised are: Does the client have the necessary prerequisite skills for this program? What training techniques have been utilized? Do alternative techniques need to be tried?

Evaluation must also occur after the IPP has been implemented. PL 94-142 requires evaluation procedures for measuring client progress on an annual basis. It is the responsibility of the IPP team to monitor the implementation of the IPP, to evaluate the effectiveness of the IPP, to identify new needs of the handicapped individual, and to evaluate the effectiveness of the IPP team. Each handicapped individual must have an annual evaluation that assesses the effectivenes of the total IPP process.

Increased Service Provider Accountability

The IPP provides considerable help in planning and providing services to handicapped individuals. Although the IPP is not a legally binding contract, it represents a statement of intent among service providers and other members of the IPP team. It specifies methodologies that will assist the handicapped individual in meeting stated goals and objectives. When members of the IPP team develop and approve the IPP, they are sanctioning the IPP as an appropriate program. This written document can prevent misunderstandings between the consumers (those receiving services) and the providers (those providing services) because it specifies individual responsibilities for implementing various components of the IPP. In addition, the IPP serves as an instructional guide to accomplishing the specified goals and objectives.

Improved Communication with Consumers

A major benefit of the IPP planning process is the involvement of the consumers. The consumers are those individuals who receive services: the handicapped individual, his/her parents and/or guardians, and advocates for the handicapped individual. By having consumers involved in the IPP process, service providers are demonstrating a concern for the outcomes of the IPP process and a concern for the needs of the consumers. The IPP communicates what specific services are to be provided to the handicapped individual rather than a general statement indicating that the handicapped individual will receive special services. Additionally, the IPP communicates and specifies levels of expectations to the handicapped individual. The person is told what is expected during the next year, what vocational and educational tasks will be worked on, and what is needed to master each task. Basically, when open communication occurs between the consumers and providers and responsibilities are shared, both groups will benefit in providing appropriate services to handicapped individuals. The IPP process has the potential for improving the quality of services provided to all handicapped individuals.

Exercise

5-1. Individualized Program Plans can improve training and service delivery in a variety of ways. List six areas that can be improved.

Answer to Exercise

5-1. 1. Coordination of planning and programming.
      2. Development of a sequential plan.
      3. Specification of individual needs and services.
      4. Systematic evaluation.
      5. Increased professional accountability.
      6. Improved communication with consumers.

COMPONENTS OF AN INDIVIDUALIZED PROGRAM PLAN

An IPP should include the following:

1. Present level of performance. This includes present academic achievement, social adaptation, prevocational and vocational skills, communication skills, and self-help skills.
2. Annual goals. These describe the performance of the individual to be achieved by the end of the year under the IPP.
3. Short-term instructional objectives. These are measurable and sequential intermediate steps between the individual's present level of performance and the annual goals.
4. Specific services needed. These services are to be determined without regard to cost or availability. The services include all services that are needed to meet the unique needs of the client.
5. Projected dates when services will be initiated and the length of time they will be provided.
6. Justification for the type of placement and services that the individual will receive.
7. Specification of the individuals who are responsible for implementation of the IPP.
8. Evaluation procedures, schedules, and objective criteria for determining whether the goals and short-term objectives were achieved. The evaluation must occur at least once a year.

There is no specified format for the development of the IPP. State and local agencies are allowed to develop their own preferred format as long as the IPPs include all of the required components. Many state and local agencies have included additional data that have expanded the IPP, such as:

1. A procedural checklist for documenting the IPP process.
2. A daily and/or weekly client schedule.
3. A list of IPP committee members.
4. Relevant test information and a client's strengths/needs list.
5. Medical information.

IPP Summary Sheet for Initial and/or 3-Month Plan[a]

NAME _____ BIRTHDATE _____

CONFERENCE PARTICIPANTS:

Name	Title	Name	Title
1.		5.	
2.		6.	
3.		7.	
4.		8.	

LIST OF ASSESSMENT INSTRUMENTS REVIEWED IN CONFERENCE:

Date Given

1. _____
2. _____
3. _____
4. _____
5. _____
6. _____
7. _____
8. _____
9. _____
10. _____

DATE FOR NEXT REVIEW _____

INDIVIDUAL _____ DATE _____

PARENT/GUARDIAN _____ DATE _____

CASE MANAGER _____ DATE _____

Strengths	Needs (Prioritized)	Action Code [b]
	1.	
	2.	
	3.	
	4.	
	5.	
	6.	
	7.	
	8.	
	9.	
	10.	
	11.	
	12.	
	13.	
	14.	

GOALS (1 year):

1. _____
2. _____
3. _____
4. _____
5. _____

(continued)

81

IPP Summary Sheet (*continued*)

FACILITIES, AND/OR PROGRAMS TO BE OFFERED:

1. _____   3. _____
2. _____   4. _____

OBJECTIVES SELECTED FOR THIS PERIOD:	DEVELOP- MENTAL AREAS[c]	PERSON RESPONSIBLE	DATE TO START	DATE TO COMPLETE
A. Prevocational				
1.				
2.				
3.				
B. Community living/residential (adaptive behavior)				
1.				
2.				
3.				
C. Health, academics and other				
1.				
2.				
3.				
4.				
5.				
6.				
7.				
8.				

[a] Developed by the Black Hills Workshop, Rapid City, South Dakota. Used by permission.

[b] Action Code: A = Is being worked on; B = No formal action to be taken at this time; C = Referred to outside agency.

[c] Key for Developmental Areas: S & E = Social and Emotional; C/A = Cognitive/Academic; S/M = Sensorimotor; C = Communicative.

6. Special materials and equipment.
7. Graphs to chart the individual's progress in meeting objectives.

A sample IPP form is included on pages 80–82.

IPP DEVELOPMENT:
OPERATIONALIZING TERMS, CONDITIONS, AND CRITERIA

Operationalized Terms

When developing the IPP it is necessary to develop long-term or annual goals and short-term objectives. Both the goals and objectives need to be stated in operationalized terms. Operationalized terms are observable and measurable descriptions of the behavior that is expected to be accomplished. For example, the statements "Sue will know her address" and "Jack will improve his vocational skills" are not operationalized descriptions of behavioral outcomes. It is hard to tell what knowing an address is or how much improvement is required.

Operationalizing behaviors is not a difficult task. It requires the instructor to describe what the client must do when the objective is accomplished. Terminology used that is open to many interpretations includes:

to know	to understand
to learn	to synthesize
to improve	to work
to comprehend	to do

Examples of operationalized terms, which are open to few interpretations, include:

to complete	to operate
to define	to name
to identify	to count
to recite	to give three reasons why

In writing operationalized goals and objectives, the criteria for acceptable performance must be considered. These criteria include important conditions, difficulty level, time, frequency, rate, and accuracy.

Important Conditions   Important conditions refer to the special circumstances surrounding the performance. In general, they reflect the who, what, when, and where of the objective.

Who—Teacher gives cue
    With the aid of a tutor
    With the group
What—Using the radial arm saw
    Using pencil and paper
    Provided with flash cards

When—When asked by the teacher
    When told to
    When given 50 items to sort
Where—In the shop
    At the group home
    In the discussion group

For example, when writing an objective the intent of which is to have a handicapped individual shake hands with a stranger, it is important to specify that shaking hands should be done when the handicapped individual is introduced to someone. Otherwise, the individual may spend his or her entire day on the corner greeting thousands of strangers as they pass by. Or, if the intent of the objective is to have a person cut a 2 × 4 board into a 6-foot length, it is important to specify whether this is to be accomplished on a table saw, radial arm saw, circular saw, or hand saw. This is because each saw is operated differently with different safety procedures.

Difficulty Level   Oftentimes when writing an operationalized goal or objective it is necessary to specify the difficulty level of the task. For example, in teaching reading skills it is necessary to state the difficulty level of the material covered, whether it is a list of survival words, Distar Reading Program Level I, or a third grade basal reader. The same is true when teaching addition. It may be necessary to state whether the individual will be working on single-digit or double-digit problems, or whether the problems require carrying skills. The difficulty level refines goals and objectives by specifying on what material mastery is expected.

Time, Frequency, Rate, and Accuracy   After the important conditions and difficulty level have been specified, it is necessary to state the acceptable criteria for mastery. The most common criteria include time, frequency, rate, and accuracy. Specifying the criteria of mastery allows you to know if the individual has accomplished an objective. Time is often used as a criterion of acceptable performance. A handicapped individual who is able to wash dishes after a dinner meal and clean the kitchen would still not have mastered these tasks if it took 4 hours to complete them. Examples of time criteria include:

1. Will remain at work station for 20 minutes.
2. Will make bed within 15 minutes.
3. Will comply with directions within 20 seconds.
4. Will mop the kitchen floor in 20 minutes.

Another criterion is frequency. Frequency refers to a count. This count may be the number of steps completed on a task analysis or the number of objects produced. If a long-term objective was for the individual to master 60 steps or components of an independent living skills curriculum, the quarterly short-term objectives may require mastery of 20, 30, 50, and finally 60 components of the program.

Often the frequency criterion is combined with a time criterion. This results in a rate criterion. Rate is frequency divided by amount of time. Suppose an agency is producing pallets. The competitive production rate for nonhandicapped individuals is 20 pallets per hour. A handicapped individual within the agency produces 20 pallets in 4 hours. This person's rate of pallet production is 5 pallets per hour (20 pallets divided by 4 hours equals 5 pallets/

hour). A potential objective for this individual would be to increase rate of pallet production from 5 pallets per hour to 20 pallets per hour.

Other ways of expressing rate criteria include:

1. Will complete 5 addition problems within 1 minute.
2. Will complete 10 situps within 1 minute.
3. Will name 10 colored flashcards within 30 seconds.
4. Will complete 10 circuit boards within 1 week.

Probably the most common and most abused criterion is accuracy. Accuracy is usually expressed in terms of a percentage, or x out of y trials—for example, "Will complete 50 math problems at 80% accuracy," or "Will correctly assemble the circuit board four out of five times." Accuracy criteria often become abused on many tasks because most tasks need to be maintained at 100% mastery. If you are going to teach a new skill or task it is important to teach the skill at 100% accuracy. If an individual is allowed an 80% accuracy level in making change from a $10 bill, we are basically saying that money is not that important and everything will work out by itself. Imagine going to a store and having an 80% chance of receiving the correct change from your purchase! Even though there is a potential for some benefit (receiving too much change back) most individuals would not frequent that store. Furthermore, no store owner would be expected to hire a cashier who displayed 80% accuracy in making change.

The same is true when the goals are stated in terms of mastery for x out of y trials. One goal written for an individual was that he would learn to cross the street correctly four out of five times. It is uncomfortable to think of what happened on the fifth attempt.

Exercise
5-2. What are operationalized terms? List and give an example of the criteria for acceptable performance that may be incorporated into an operationalized definition of behavior.

Answer to Exercise
5-2. Operationalized terms are observable and measurable descriptions of behavior. In writing operationalized goals and objectives, criteria that may be incorporated include important conditions, difficulty level, time, frequency, rate, and accuracy.

LONG-TERM OBJECTIVES OR ANNUAL GOALS

The long-term objectives form the outline of the IPP. They are what the IPP team has agreed to work on during the upcoming year. Thompson (1977) indicated that appropriate long-term objectives have five components:

1. Direction of change.
2. Statement of deficit or excess.
3. A "from" statement.
4. A "to" statement.
5. Resources needed.

Direction

Direction of change refers to what is to be accomplished with the individual's behavior. There are only three things that can be done with a behavior: it can be increased, maintained, or decreased. For example, one can:

Increase—attention to work, the number of pallets completed, recognition of survival words, number of steps completed on a task analysis.
Maintain—rate of pallet production, dressing skills, being able to buy groceries for one week's meals, attention to work.
Decrease—number of temper tantrums, number of math errors, days absent, the amount of time required to get dressed.

When working with handicapped individuals, most of the long-term goals should be directed at increasing behaviors. This is because it is the function of the agency to bring these individuals to higher levels of performance, and behaviors increase as a result of positive reinforcement procedures. How the long-term objective is written determines which behavior change technique is to be utilized. Since we want to increase the level of performance, positive reinforcement techniques are called for.

Statement of Deficit or Excess

The statement of deficit or excess refers to the behavior that needs to be changed. *Deficits in behaviors* means there are behaviors that do not occur frequently enough and/or for which the client does not have the prerequisite skills. Deficits therefore refer to behaviors that are to be increased or improved. Examples of behaviors in which deficits can occur include:

1. Rate of pallet production.
2. Fine motor skills.
3. Attending to task.
4. Following directions.
5. Number of steps completed on a task analysis.

Excessive behaviors are behaviors that occur too frequently. Excessive behaviors are behaviors that are to be decreased. Examples of excessive behaviors include:

1. Incidents of physical aggressiveness.
2. Noncompliance.
3. Not attending to task.

4. Number of errors made on math assignments.
5. Number of times person leaves work station.

There are two ways to approach behavior problems. The first way requires implementation of a program designed to decrease behaviors. The second requires a behavioral program designed to increase the periods of time between undesirable behaviors. For example, one way to deal with temper tantrums is to decrease the number of tantrums and the other is to increase the amount of time between tantrums. The second approach requires the use of positive reinforcement techniques and builds on the client's strengths, which is the preferred approach.

"From" Statement

The "from" statement is a description of the individual's present level of functioning within the area of deficit or excess. Examples of "from" statements include:

1. From building 2 pallets per hour.
2. From completing six steps of the task analysis.
3. From being dressed with physical assistance.
4. From being able to stack two blocks.
5. From leaving the work station four times per hour.

"To" Statement

The "to" statement refers to the expected level of performance after the remedial program has been implemented. In general, it reflects the goal to be attained at the end of the upcoming year. Examples of "to" statements include:

1. To build 15 pallets per hour.
2. To complete all steps of the task analysis.
3. To only leave the work station with permission.
4. To name the numbers 1 through 10 when presented with flashcards.
5. To comply with instructions within 5 seconds of being given them.

Resources Needed

Not all goals will require a statement regarding resources that are needed to accomplish the objective. However, many objectives require a statement regarding what resources will be needed to accomplish the expected level of performance. The resources may be specialists, materials, and methods. Resource statements include:

1. Use of speech therapy.
2. Use of Distar Reading Series.
3. Use of individual counseling.
4. Use of vocational rehabilitation services.

In summary,

Statement of Direction + Statement of Deficit/Excess + "From" Statement + "To" Statement + Resources Needed = Long-term Objectives

    Joe will increase his dressing skills from being dressed with physical assistance to being able to dress independently by using the independent living curriculum.

SHORT-TERM OBJECTIVES

Short-term objectives are the intermediate steps between the client's present levels of functioning and the expected levels of functioning stated in the long-term objectives. They specify intermediate steps between the "from" and "to" statements. Short-term objectives are operationalized descriptions of the intended outcomes of intervention strategies. They include the criteria by which intervention success is to be measured. Operationalized statements noting important conditions, difficulty level, and time, frequency, and accuracy criteria are also included. Short-term objectives provide a way of evaluating how the individual is progressing on programs and how well programs are working. Short-term objectives may include:

1. Operationalized terms.
2. Methodology.
3. Levels of performance.
4. Special resources.
5. Criteria of acceptable performance.

Operationalized Terms

Remember, operationalized terms are descriptions of behaviors that are observable and measurable. Two instructors observing the same client engaged in a behavior that has been operationally defined will be able to agree on the occurrence or nonoccurrence of that particular behavior. The operationalized behavior should reflect the intended outcome of the intervention strategy. As mentioned earlier, terms such as to learn, to improve, and to know are ambiguous, and can lead to misinterpretations by various IPP team members. Operationalized terms are descriptors that are limited to few interpretations.

Methodology

Methodology refers to who will do what, where, and when—in other words, how the long-term objective will be accomplished. It is necessary to specify procedures that staff are to implement in order to accomplish these objectives. The methodology is usually written as a teaching plan or an objective plan. A sample objective plan is included on page 89.

OBJECTIVE PLAN[a]

CLIENT: _____
PROGRAM/AREA: _____
GOAL (1 Year): _____

DATE PROGRAM STARTED: _____
EXPECTED DATE OF COMPLETION: _____

OBJECTIVE: _____

PRESENT BASELINE BEHAVIOR: _____

RESPONSIBLE STAFF/PERSON: _____

PROGRAM EVENTS AND/OR METHODS

ACCELERATION OF BEHAVIOR		DECELERATION OF BEHAVIOR
Reinforcer		Contingency

EVALUATION
CRITERIA:
1) Accomplished objective _____
2) Partial completion of 50% or more _____
3) Reasons for not accomplishing objective
   A) Lack of resources such as: _____
   B) Need to try other methods such as: _____
   C) Other barriers: _____

[a]Developed by the Black Hills Workshop, Rapid City, South Dakota. Used by permission.

As was the case with long-term objectives, it is necessary to use operationalized statements when writing out specific methodologies. Statements such as "Joe will work with Sally on prevocational training from 9:30 to 11:30, three days a week" are not operationalized statements, because there is no mention of what is to be taught or how it will be taught during prevocational training. An appropriate teaching/objective plan is constructed so that any staff member can read the plan and implement the program correctly, even if the staff member has had no prior experience with the program. Specific consideration needs to be given to scheduling and instructions and cues.

Scheduling   When selecting program methodologies it is necessary to allocate resources (staff, materials) to accomplish objectives. Types of questions that need to be addressed include: How many behaviors should be worked on at one time? Should the program be designed to increase fine motor skills, attention span, or both? Should the program be designed to decrease temper tantrums, noncompliance, yelling, and throwing objects, or should the program attempt to decrease only one of these behaviors?

It is easy to become overwhelmed with the number of deficits in behavior and excessive behaviors that are exhibited by handicapped individuals. Often agency staff attempt to work on too many behaviors and staff resources are stretched beyond reasonable limits. The best philosophy is to program for a small number of new behaviors at a time and, once progress is seen on these behaviors, then add more. Use small steps in your programs. If the client is not progressing it is the fault of your program, *not* the client's fault. Additional considerations include: How many staff should be involved in the program? What is the intensity of the program? What is the client's past learning history?

Instructions and Cues   When training programs are implemented, staff use instructions and cues to communicate desired behaviors to the client. The most common errors made with *verbal cues* are that staff use vocabulary the client does not understand, overly complex instructions, too many repetitions, or verbalizations that are too long. In communicating instructions to a client it is not always necessary to say, "Sally, I want you to go over to the coat rack and select your coat from the others that are hanging up. Your coat is the blue one that comes to your thighs and has a zipper. It also has a hood and a pale blue lining with fur around the collar." Often a simple statement such as "Sally, please get your coat" will do. Additionally, many staff believe that, if a client does not follow instructions the first time, repeating the instructions in a much louder voice will somehow make the client comply with the request.

When using verbal cues, consider: vocabulary used, complexity of instructions, length of verbalization, vocal components (volume, tone), and repetitions or restatements.

If a staff member does not communicate instructions with appropriate *nonverbal cues,* learning is often impeded. The amount of learning that takes place when a staff member yells at a client from across the room is questionable. Furthermore, the attitude expressed when staff give instructions without looking at the client says much about the amount of effort that the client will exhibit when complying with the instructions.

When using nonverbal cues, consider: eye contact, smiling, laughing, facial gestures, body motions, physical contact, and level of attention before giving the cue.

Training cues are those cues that are related to the specific behaviors that are to be taught. They may refer to the different sizes of objects to be assembled or to a picture of materials needed. Training cues serve as discriminative stimuli, which are one of the bases of learning (see Chapter 7).

When using training cues, consider: type of cue, number of cues, proximity to client, distinctive features (size, texture, shape, color, weight), complexity of cue, and novelty of cue.

General cues refer to environmental cues that set the occasion for certain client behaviors to occur. For example, when in the community residence program, it is alright to leave your chair and go to the kitchen to make popcorn. At work, however, this behavior would not be tolerated. In other words, the client must discriminate between work and leisure time.

When using general cues, consider:

1. Physical setting
   a. Seating position
   b. Job task
2. General rules
   a. Rules and policies
   b. Expectations of staff
   c. Consistency level
   d. Staff reminders/reprimands
3. Physical layout
   a. Visual distractions
   b. Auditory distractions
4. Social factors
   a. Work or recreation
   b. Other client behavior
   c. Others receiving attention
   d. Friendship factors

In summary, the instructions and cues given by staff serve as discriminative stimuli. Discriminative stimuli set the occasion for certain behaviors to occur. When teaching new behaviors, it is essential to maximize the use of the instructions and cues given. Further discussion of discriminative stimuli is provided in Chapters 7 and 9.

Levels of Performance

Levels of performance specify the criteria for and conditions in which training is to occur. Consideration must be given to the setting of the training session. For example, is training to occur on a one-to-one basis or a group basis? In a quiet room or in the production area? Additional thought should be given to whether the present setting is related to possible future settings or other similar situations.

Other levels of performance should address the client's abilities in mastering the task, and specifically the client's response to prompts. Prompts are levels of assistance provided by the instructor. Prompts may be physical, gestural, or verbal in nature. Physical prompts are those in which staff physically assist the client in accomplishing a task or behavior. A staff member might provide a physical prompt in teaching a client to sweep a floor by standing behind the client and placing his or her hands over the client's hands while grasping a broom. This prompt might continue with the staff member assisting in several "sweeps."

A gestural prompt requires less physical assistance to the client. The staff member provides a gesture to assist the client in accomplishing the task or the behavior. For sweeping, the staff member might point to the broom or might make a sweeping motion with his or her hands and arms to assist the client.

A verbal prompt provides no physical assistance to the client. Rather, the staff member gives verbal cues to the client that will assist the client in completing the task or the behavior. For sweeping, the staff member may provide verbal prompts such as "get the broom" or "sweep over there."

The level of prompt is specified in the methodology so that the instructor will know how much physical or verbal assistance is to be provided to the client in order for the client to accomplish the task or a specific behavior. Ultimately, the client will be able to perform the task independently or with minimal verbal prompts.

Special Resources

When specifying the procedures that are to be utilized it is necessary to identify which staff members are to be responsible for accomplishing certain tasks. Additionally, special materials and resources need to be identified. If a staff member is to instruct a client in money identification, it is necessary to specify whether a certain task analysis is to be utilized, whether real or play money is to be used, or whether a prepackaged program is to be utilized. Other special resources include whether or not certain jigs, braces, containers, materials, or numerous other apparatus or materials are to be used during the training program.

Criteria

Criteria of acceptable performance are used to determine whether the objective has been accomplished. As mentioned earlier, these criteria may include time, frequency, rate, difficulty level, and/or accuracy, depending on the objective.

Exercises

5-3. List and describe the five components of a long-term objective.
5-4. Define a short-term objective and describe five components of short-term objectives.
5-5. Write an appropriate long-term and short-term objective for the following:

Carol is participating in a residential training program. A need is identified for Carol to be able to walk to the work activity center independently. When Carol was asked to walk to the center, she walked out of the house, waited, and then sat on the porch steps. The work activities center is eight blocks away from the house.

Answers to Exercises

5-3.   1. Direction of change—whether the behavior is to be increased, decreased, or maintained.

        2. Statement of deficit or excess—deficits in behavior imply the behaviors are to be increased, while excessive behaviors are to be decreased. The majority of programming should emphasize increasing or improving desirable client behaviors.

        3. "From" statement—based on current levels of performance.

        4. "To" statement—reflects where the client will be within 1 year of when the goal is written.

        5. Resources needed—required special resources are identified.

5-4. Short-term objectives are the sequential steps between the client's present level of functioning and the expected level of functioning specified in the "to" statement of the long-term objective. Short-term objectives should include: 1) operationalized terms, 2) specific methodologies, 3) specified levels of performance, 4) special resources, and 5) criteria of acceptable performance.

5-5.   1. *Long-term objective.* Carol will increase her community orientation skills from not being able to independently walk from the group home to the work activity center to independently walking to the work activity center from the group home.

        2. *Short-term objective I.* Carol will walk independently the last four blocks to the work activity center (WAC) when it is time to go to work. A staff member (John or Jan) will tell Carol that it is time to go to work and will walk with Carol to the work activity center. The staff member will walk Carol to one-half, one, one-and-a-half, and two blocks away from the WAC. Carol must walk independently the remaining distance for three consecutive days before the distance is increased.

        3. *Short-term objective II.* Carol will be told to go to work and walk independently to the WAC from two-and-a-half, three, four, and five blocks away. Carol must walk independently to the WAC for three consecutive days before the distance is increased.

        4. *Short-term objective III.* Carol will continue to be told to go to work and will walk independently to the WAC from six, seven, and eight blocks away. She must walk independently to the WAC for three consecutive days before the distance is increased.

        5. *Short-term objective IV.* Carol will walk independently from the group home to the WAC. She will be told to walk to work, but the staff member will not walk with her.

SUMMARY

The Individualized Program Plan assists professionals in planning and providing services to handicapped individuals. Although there is no standardized form for an Individualized Program Plan, the minimum components should include statements regarding:

1. Present level of performance.
2. Annual goals or long-term goals.
3. Short-term goals.
4. Specific services needed.
5. Projected dates when special services will be initiated.
6. Justification for the type of placement and services needed.
7. Specification of the individuals who are responsible for the implementation of the IPP.
8. Evaluation procedures, schedules, and objective criteria for determining whether the long-term and short-term objectives were achieved.

The long-term objectives reflect where the individual should be within 1 year of beginning the program. Each long-term objective should consist of:

1. Direction of change.
2. A statement of deficit or excess.
3. A "from" statement.
4. A "to" statement.
5. Resources needed.

The short-term objectives reflect a sequential progression from the handicapped individual's present level of performance to the long-term objective. Short-term objectives should consist of:

1. Operationalized terms.
2. Methodology.
3. Levels of performance.
4. Special resources.
5. Criteria of acceptable performance.

The long-term objective and short-term objective are derived from the handicapped individual's assessment and IPP process. It is necessary to know where the individual is prior to setting long-term objectives. Additionally, the short-term objectives must reflect sequential steps between the individual's present level of functioning and his or her expected level of functioning. There must be a direct logical relationship between the short-term objectives and the long-term objective. The long-term objective should reflect the sum of all of its short-term objectives.

Operationalized Terms	+	Important Conditions	+	Criteria of Mastery	=	Short-term Objective

Short-Term Objective I

Bill will independently complete steps
1 through 8 of the toothbrushing
task analysis at 100% accuracy.

+

Short-Term Objective II

Bill will independently complete steps
1 through 10.

+

Short-Term Objective III

Bill will independently complete steps 1
through 14.

+

Short-Term Objective IV

Bill will independently complete steps
1 through 16.

=

Long-Term Objective

Bill will increase his toothbrushing skills
from independently completing steps 1
through 4 of the toothbrushing task
analysis to independently completing all
16 steps of the toothbrushing task analysis.

Effective client programming is the result of the IPP process. Although developing an IPP may appear tedious, once you become familiar with the process the amount of time required to develop an IPP decreases and training becomes more efficient. For example, prior to the annual IPP staffing, team members should prepare a list of client strengths, needs, and possible goal areas.

The authors utilize an IPP procedural checklist when working with IPP teams to identify the team's strengths and needs. A sample is included on pages 96–97. The entire IPP is comprised of the following process:

1. Involve the client.
2. List client's strengths.
3. List client's needs.
4. List and prioritize goals to be worked on.
5. Suggest and prioritize strategies that will be used to increase behaviors that are currently client deficits. Review strength list to see if client's strengths may be used to work on client's needs.
6. Develop the IPP by writing appropriate long-term and short-term objectives for each client goal.

Observation/Critique of Goal Planning

CLIENT: _____ REVIEWER: _____

FACILITY: _____ DATE: _____

I. Critical elements of goal planning:
   A. Involve client
   B. Use strengths to help with needs
   C. Use small steps
   D. Set target dates
   F. State what client and staff will do

II. Staff Strengths

    (What was done right and what was
    done especially well)

    Staff Needs

    (State positively; i.e., what staff
    could do to improve goal planning)

III. Documentation
   A. Are background data (including strengths/needs list) adequate to understand the client's program?
      Comments:

   B. Are goal plans completed and clearly filled out?
      1. Clear language? Yes _____ No _____
         Comments:

      2. Goals stated in terms of client behavior? Yes _____ No _____
         Comments:

      3. Staff responsibilities clearly stated and responsible staff named?
         Yes _____ No _____
         Comments:

Observation/Critique of Goal Planning (*continued*)

4. Target date for current steps in goal plan? Yes _____ No _____
Comments:

IV. Interactions with Client
   A. Was the client maximally involved?
      1. Did he or she participate in choosing the goals?
         Yes _____ No _____
         Comments:

      2. Was he or she given choice in the plans? Yes _____ No _____
         Comments:

      3. Were the plans explained to him or her? Yes _____ No _____
         Comments:

   B. If the client could not actively participate, did the staff include his or her likes and wants in the plan? Yes _____ No _____
      Comments:

V. Other Comments
   A. Do you have any suggestions about the goals or methods for staff to consider?

   B. Staff comments and self-critique:

   C. Recommendations to improve these problems:

SUGGESTED ACTIVITIES

1. Identify ways in which your IPP process has improved training and service delivery.
2. Review a client's long-term and short-term objectives. Are they related to the client's needs? Do they incorporate the essential components of objective writing?
3. Utilize the observation sheets in Figure 5-3 to critique a goal-planning meeting at your facility. Identify deficits of the meeting and design a program to increase desired behaviors.

ADDITIONAL RESOURCES

Houts, P. S., & Scott, R. A. *Goal planning for the developmentally disabled.* Hershey, Penna.: Pennsylvania State University, 1975.

Houts, P. S., & Scott, R. A. *Help! I've got a problem. Goal planning strategies for difficult client behaviors.* Hershey, Penna.: Pennsylvania State University, 1976. (a)

Houts, P. S., & Scott, R. A. *New direction without insurrection.* Hershey, Penna.: Pennsylvania State University, 1976. (b)

Lynn, J. J., Waltz, D., & Brush, W. *The individual educational program (IEP) manual.* Hollister, Calif.: Argonaut Publications, 1977.

REFERENCES

Carroll, L. *Alice's adventures in Wonderland.* Springfield, Mass.: McLaughlin Brothers Inc.

Thompson, D. G. *Writing long-term and short-term objectives.* Champaign, Ill.: Research Press, 1977.

Turnbull, A. P., Strickland, B. B., & Brantley, J. C. *Developing and implementing individualized education programs.* Columbus, Ohio: Charles E. Merrill, 1978.

Unit III

Behavioral Assessment
Where Are We?

Chapter 6

Measuring, Recording, and Reporting Behavior

OBJECTIVES

To be able to:

1. Give three reasons for measuring behavior.
2. Give operational definitions for behaviors to be measured.
3. List and define the measurable dimensions of behavior.
4. List and define three approaches to recording behavior.
5. List the types of instrumentation for measuring behavior and the measurement approaches for which each is used.
6. Give three answers to the question of who measures.
7. List possible reactions to observation by the observer and by those being observed.
8. Give the reason for checking observer agreement.
9. Calculate observer agreement.
10. List advantages and disadvantages of self-monitoring.
11. Report data in graphic and tabular form.
12. Design measurement procedures that operationally define behavior and tell who will measure it, when, how, and where.

MEASURING BEHAVIOR

Why Measure?

Many people react negatively to our suggestions that they measure client behavior. We are often told that staff already have too much paperwork to do, and that taking data will reduce time spent working with clients. To some extent these are reasonable objections. Measuring behavior does mean more paperwork, and sometimes reduces client contact time. However, there are simple ways to measure behavior that require little time and minimal paperwork. More important, there are some excellent reasons for measuring behavior that you are interested in changing. They are:

1. *Human judgments of what someone does are frequently inaccurate (Kazdin, 1975).* We often are told that a client has temper tantrums all the time, only to find that the tantrums in fact occur once or twice a week. On the other hand, staff often become so used to a mildly irritating behavior that the behavior is seen as happening infrequently even though it really occurs several times a day.

2. *We need to measure behavior to know whether we are justified in trying to change it (Martin & Pear, 1978).* A severely handicapped man was once referred to one of the authors for a program designed to increase his attention to his work. Careful measurement showed that he was already on task 95% of the time! As a result, everyone's time was used more profitably to work on problems that really were problems instead of trying to solve a problem that didn't exist.

3. *Measurements of behavior can be useful in choosing an intervention strategy (Martin & Pear, 1978).* We need to carefully identify what is happening so that we can make a guess about what is controlling a behavior and therefore decide how to change it. This type of assessment is known as a *functional analysis of behavior (Gardner, 1971).*

4. *We have to know where we are in order to decide whether we've gone anywhere (Martin & Pear, 1978).* If you don't measure what clients are doing before you start a program, measurements of their behavior after you start will be meaningless because you won't have any way to make a comparison. This is why baseline data are so important. Baseline data are preprogram measures of behavior (Kazdin, 1975). You should collect them before beginning any program.

5. *Publicly displayed data can reinforce staff for carrying out programs and therefore increase the likelihood that they will continue to do so (Martin & Pear, 1978).* This makes good sense—we are all more likely to keep doing something we're supposed to do if we can see that it is having the effect we want or if we know that other people are aware of what we're doing. In one institution, the number of training sessions conducted by staff increased substantially after the psychologist started posting feedback sheets showing the number of sessions conducted out of the total number scheduled (Panyan, Boozer, & Morris, 1970).

6. *Posted data can also reinforce clients for behavior change (Martin & Pear, 1978).* A colorful graph showing an increase in work productivity can be used to encourage continued high production. Even severely handicapped persons can understand clearly, creatively designed visual feedback. For example, if the person is working toward earning enough money to make a large purchase, a picture of the item to be purchased

can be cut up like a jigsaw puzzle and a piece added every time a set amount is earned.

7. *Measuring client behavior increases our accountability.* It tells us and the public whether we are having the effects we want to have on those we serve. It is absolutely critical that we be accountable for what we do; otherwise we will lose public and financial support for our services. This is because "Many people are no longer content to accept methods that are used simply because the practitioner is trained to use them, because he has a strong intuitive feeling that they will work, or because the student, client, or an informal observer reports that they work" (Sulzer & Mayer, 1972, p. 262).

Exercise

6-1. Give at least three reasons for measuring behavior.

Answers to Exercise

6-1. Any three of the following:
   a. Human judgments of behavior are often not accurate.
   b. Measuring behavior helps us to know whether we should change it.
   c. Measurements can be useful in choosing an intervention strategy.
   d. We must know where we are in order to know whether we've gone anywhere.
   e. Publicly displayed data can reinforce staff for carrying out programs.
   f. Publicly displayed data can reinforce clients for behavior change.
   g. Measuring client behavior increases accountability.

What to Measure

Too often staff using behavior change procedures decide on a procedure, start measuring behavior, and start the program without ever performing a careful functional analysis of the behavior. A functional analysis involves identifying the antecedents and consequences related to problem behaviors. Antecedents are events that occur just before problem behaviors, and consequences are events that follow problem behaviors (Keefe, Kopel, & Gordon, 1978).

One good way to begin a functional analysis is to take anecdotal records. Anecdotal records are written descriptions of the behavior of interest, as well as antecedents and consequences. They should also include a specific description of the conditions under which the behavior occurs: who is present, time, place, and nature of task or activity (Haywood, Filler, Shifman, & Chatelanat, 1975).

Perhaps the two most difficult things to learn about taking useful anecdotal records are to be specific and to avoid making judgments. Writing "the supervisor praised her work" is not specific; writing "the supervisor said 'Good job, Nancy' " is specific. Writing "he was angry" is making a judgment; writing "he called me a liar and threw the knife at me" is a good description.

At the end of this chapter (page 128), a blank sample of a form used to record anecdotal descriptions of behavior is included. Figure 6-1 provides an example of a good anecdotal record obtained using this form. Notice that the record tells you what Joe did. This information is much more important than describing what Joe did not do (Gardner, 1977). When we are told that Joe's problem is "not working," our immediate response is always to ask what he is doing. Only if we know what someone is doing can we identify and then change whatever factors are maintaining the behavior.

Operational Definitions of Behavior

You have to identify the behavior to be observed before you take anecdotal records, but at this stage it is difficult to specifically define the behavior. Once you have anecdotal descriptions, then you can define the behavior in specific

		Anecdotal Record Form		
Client __Joe Blow__ Observer __Jim Supervisor__ Date ___10/21___				
Time	Antecedents	Behavior	Consequences	Location
9:00 A.M.	I say "Get to work, Joe."	Joe begins assembling curtain rods.		shop
9:10 A.M.	Visiting psychologist walks in	Joe puts down work, walks over to her and says, "Hi, how are you?"	She says "Fine."	
9:11 A.M.	I say "Get back to work, Joe."	Joe goes ck to work.		
9:30 A.M.	I start coughing.	Joe gets up, comes over to me, pats my back.	I say "Back to work, Joe."	
9:31 A.M.	I say "Back to work, Joe."	Joe goes back to work.		
9:45 A.M.	Other clients going on break.	Joe continues working.	I say "Joe, time for break."	
9:46 A.M.	I say "Joe, time for break."	Joe leaves for break.		

Figure 6-1. Anecdotal record of Joe's behavior. Notice that the record tells exactly what Joe did, not what he did not do.

or operational terms. An operational definition is one that uses *observable and measurable terms* (Keefe et al., 1978).

In order for a definition to be observable, it must describe not only the behavior to be observed, but also the conditions under which it occurs. Specifically, your definition should include who is doing what, how, where, and when (Gardner, 1971). Two examples of operational definitions are:

Who: Joan
What: going on break independently
Where: adjustment training center
When: 10:15, noon, 2:30 M–F
How: stop work at break times, leave work station, go to restroom and/or break room

Who: Tim
What: answering telephone
Where: group home living room
When: whenever phone rings
How: pick up receiver, hold to ear with mouthpiece at mouth, say "hello"

After you have agreed on an operational definition and taken some baseline data on the defined behavior, you may find you need to revise your definition. There are three reasons definitions may need revision. Perhaps the most common reason is that the definition is too vague, and your staff are therefore not all observing the same behavior (Sulzer & Mayer, 1972). A typical flaw in definitions is that they include the word "appropriate." For instance, "greeting strangers appropriately" is not an operationally defined behavior, and it is unlikely that all the staff at your agency have precisely the same definition of "appropriately." The only way around this is to sit down and agree on how to describe appropriate greetings so that everyone will be able to identify them.

Another reason you may need to review a definition is that you may be observing the wrong behavior. Remember that the reason for operationally defining and measuring a behavior is so that you can tell if it changes. If you find yourself defining a behavior that does not need to be changed, i.e., that is not related to your client's goals, forget about it and define a different, goal-related behavior. For instance, you may be observing how much a person is attending to a task when the goal for that person is not to increase time on task, but to increase production rate. Therefore, you should be observing production rate, not time on task.

Finally, you may want to revise a definition to make it proactive. We often begin to describe behaviors in terms of excesses: the client does too much of something. Although one of our goals may be to reduce the occurrence of a behavior, we should also know what we want the individual to do instead. Decreasing excesses is reactive whereas increasing positive behaviors or teaching new ones is proactive. If Mary displays an excess of leaving her work station, she has a deficit in staying there. Teaching her to stay at the work station is proactive.

Dimensions of Behavior

There are five dimensions of behavior that you may wish to measure. The first, and most commonly used, is *frequency*. Frequency refers to how many times a behavior occurs while you are observing it (Martin & Pear, 1978). For instance, if you are interested in how many assembly units an individual completes, you are interested in frequency.

Before you can compare frequencies obtained across several different observation periods, you may need to convert the frequencies to *rates*. Rate is defined as frequency divided by length of time of observation. The reason for converting frequencies to rates is that, when observation periods are not all the same length, the frequencies you obtain are not directly comparable (Kazdin, 1975). For example, suppose the frequency with which a worker completed assembling curtain rods was observed for one working week. Suppose those frequencies were Monday—50, Tuesday—60, Wednesday—45, Thursday—30, Friday—25. This looks like production decreased at the end of the week. However, this worker was on the job for 6 hours each day on Monday, Tuesday, and Wednesday, but only 3 hours each day on Thursday and Friday. Therefore, his production rates were:

M   50 rods/6 hr. = 8.3 rods/hr.
T   60 rods/6 hr. = 10 rods/hr.
W   45 rods/6 hr. = 7.5 rods/hr.
TH 30 rods/3 hr. = 10 rods/hr.
F   25 rods/3 hr. = 8.3 rods/hr.

So, as you can see, production did not decrease at the end of the week.

Another dimension of behavior that is often measured is *duration*. Duration is a measure of how long a behavior lasts (Sulzer & Mayer, 1972). We are often interested in how long an individual works continuously on a task, how long people spend interacting with others, or how long a person goes without temper tantrums. In each case we are interested in duration.

Sometimes we want to know how long it is between the presentation of a stimulus and the beginning of the response to it. This dimension of behavior is called *latency* (Martin & Pear, 1978). It is most often measured with respect to compliance. That is, we measure the length of time between when an instruction is given and when the person starts to follow the instruction.

We also often measure the *form* of a behavior. This is a measure of accuracy: we want to know if the observed behavior meets certain standards for form. You are probably familiar with measures of form from your school days. When your math teacher recorded how many right answers you had out of the number possible on a test, he was recording your accuracy. You may be interested in recording the accuracy of such things as bed-making or work assemblies.

The fifth dimension of behavior is *intensity*. This is the most difficult dimension to measure in a natural setting because exact measures of intensity usually require laboratory equipment. If we want to measure how loudly or softly someone speaks, we are interested in intensity (Gardner, 1977). Since it is unlikely that you have sound level meters to measure intensity of volume, one alternative method is to rate speech volume as to how loud or soft it is. Three-point to five-point rating scales are most often used to measure intensity. For example, speech volume might be rated as too loud, normal range, or too soft.

Sometimes people speak of measuring the *quality* of a behavior, such as work production. Quality can be thought of as a combination of two or more dimensions of behavior. One common combination is that of rate and form (Warren, Rogers-Warren, & Baer, 1975). Suppose you are teaching an individual to make sandwiches for a picnic. The quality of sandwich-making depends on both rate and form. That is, you will want the person to make a sufficient number of sandwiches in a given time period (e.g., 10 sandwiches in 20 minutes), and you will want the sandwiches to meet certain standards for form (e.g., meat between two slices of bread, not on top of them). Whenever you are interested in the quality of a behavior, you will probably need to measure more than one dimension of behavior.

One characteristic of behavior that can relate to any of the dimensions is *variability*. If a person displays about the same rate of behavior over several observations, the behavior has low variability. However, if the person's rates are inconsistent and show large changes between observations, the behavior is highly variable, or inconsistent. Sometimes modifying variability of behavior is an important goal (Jones, 1972).

Exercises

6-2. What are the two characteristics of an operational definition?

6-3. What are the measurable dimensions of behavior?

For each of the anecdotal descriptions below (6-4 through 6-8), give an operational definition of the behavior described and tell which measurable dimension of behavior you have described.

6-4. I told Joe to set the table for dinner. Ten minutes later he finally started getting out the dishes.

6-5. Nancy walked to the curb, looked both ways, and immediately began to cross the street while the light was still red. I grabbed her to stop her.

6-6. Rhoda said hello to me 30 times this morning!

6-7. Mike said something to me during break this afternoon. I couldn't hear him even though I was standing right next to him.

6-8. Teresa only worked for an hour out of a 6-hour workday today.

6-9. Lucille cried seven times one day. What is the frequency of crying behavior for that day?

6-10. During a 10-minute observation period, Marian emitted 32 "stereotypic" behaviors. What is the rate per minute? _____

6-11. Out of 10 commands, Peter complied with 7. What is his percentage of compliance? _____

6-12. Out of 13 spelling words, Jean spelled 9 correctly during a written drill. What was her percentage correct? _____

6-13. Martha asked Rafael to come to her, which he did after 22 seconds. What is the latency of the response? _____

6-14. Give the rate for each of the following time samples from one work day and the average rate per minute for the day.

Frequency of assembling curtain rods	Observation time	Rate/minute
22	10 min.	
15	7 min.	
20	8 min.	

Average rate/minute _____

Answers to Exercises

6- 2. Observable, measurable.

6- 3. Frequency, duration, latency, form, intensity.

6- 4. The behavior is beginning to set the table by starting toward the dish cupboard. The dimension is latency.

6- 5. The behavior is stopping at the curb, looking both ways, and then crossing the street only when the light is green and no cars are coming. The dimension is accuracy.

6- 6. The behavior is saying hello to someone she has already said hello to on the same day in the same location. The dimension is frequency.

6- 7. The behavior is speaking too softly to be heard to someone no more than 2 feet away. The dimension is intensity.

6- 8. The behavior is working, which might be defined as having at least one hand on the parts to be assembled. The dimension is duration.

6- 9. 7

6-10. 3.2/min.

6-11. 70%

6-12. 69%

6-13. 22 seconds

6-14. 2.2
2.14
2.5
Average = 2.28

RECORDING BEHAVIOR

How to Record Behavior

Once you have chosen the dimension of behavior you wish to measure, you need to decide how to measure it. The most complete way to measure behavior is called *continuous event recording*. This means you record every occurrence of the behavior during a specified period. You can be recording frequency, duration, intensity, latency, form, or some combination of these variables. Event recording is usually used to measure behaviors with a clear beginning and ending (Gardner, 1977). Getting dressed and crossing the street are two such behaviors.

Another way to measure behavior is called *interval recording.* This procedure involves dividing a period of time into short, equal intervals. These intervals typically are from 10 seconds to 2 minutes long. Then, once per interval, you record whether or not the behavior you are observing occurred (Martin & Pear, 1978). This procedure is often used to measure behaviors that do not have clear beginnings and endings, or that vary in duration (Gardner, 1977). On-task behaviors, for instance, often do not have clear beginnings and endings. When someone is in the process of putting down or ceasing work on a task, it can be very difficult to determine at what precise instant they are no longer on task.

Sometimes behaviors occur so frequently that it is not practical to observe them during the entire period of interest. Self-stimulatory behaviors such as body-rocking and finger-twirling usually fit this description. In these cases *time sampling* is used to obtain a representative sample of the behaviors (Gardner, 1977). This procedure involves measuring behavior during each of several short time periods within the larger period of interest.

When you use time sampling, you want your measurements to be representative. That is, you want to get data that represent the person's behavior over the larger period of interest (Gardner, 1977). There are two ways of choosing time samples: random and systematic. To select *random time samples,* you divide the period during which the behavior of interest occurs into separate short time intervals, usually 5 to 15 minutes long. Then you decide how many samples per period you want to take and choose that many at random from the total list. Since you then choose another set at random for each period (usually a day) random time sampling is not very practical for agencies without a research staff. That is because the observation times change daily, which is very difficult to schedule.

Consequently, you will probably use *systematic time sampling.* To do so, decide how many time samples you need for each period of interest and how long each sample will be. Then systematically choose the time each sample will be taken by arranging for the samples at the various times of the day in which you are interested and in all the settings of interest.

Time samples can be used with either continuous event recording or interval recording. Thus, you have four possible ways to record behavior: (1) continuous event recording during the entire period of interest, (2) interval recording during the entire period of interest, (3) continuous event recording during time samples, and (4) interval recording during time samples. Examples of each of these possibilities are:

1. Continuous event recording during the entire period of interest—Record the length of every temper tantrum a person displays at any time. (This will give you frequency as well as duration.)
2. Interval recording during the entire period of interest—Every 2 minutes during every break and lunch period at the workshop, record whether or not an individual is talking with anyone else.
3. Continuous event recording during time samples—During each of four 30-minute samples every day, two of which are taken at the training center on weekdays, record whether a person's speech is too loud, too soft, or acceptable each time they speak.
4. Interval recording during time samples—For the first 2 minutes of every hour during the working day, record at the end of every 10 seconds whether or not an individual is on task.

Tools for Recording Behavior

The most common tools for recording behavior are paper and pencil. Obviously, measuring behavior won't help you unless you record the results so that everyone involved in programming can see them. Most recording is done on forms that have spaces for all the information needed so that you don't forget anything. Many types of standard forms are already available. Standard forms that can be used for frequency, duration, or latency measures, as well as one for interval recording, are included at the end of this chapter on pages 129–132. Illustrated on page 133 is one possible form to use in recording intensity, in this case vocal volume, while on page 134 a sample chart for recording form, in this case whether ballpoint pens have been assembled correctly, is provided.

Sometimes it is not practical to carry a pencil and paper with you during an observation period. When this is the case, you may want to use either a hand-held counter, such as the kind used to keep track of how much you spend in the grocery store, or a counter you can wear on your wrist, such as a golf counter (Gardner, 1977). Counters you can wear are particularly useful because they leave your hands free. It is also possible to wear and use more than one at a time, as long as you remember which counter you're using to record which behavior. It is easier to keep track of multiple counters if the wrist bands are each a different color or if you always wear them in the same order.

You will always need a clock or watch in order to record when you began observations and when you finished them. In addition, if you are measuring latency of behavior or a behavior of brief duration, you will need a stopwatch (Sulzer & Mayer, 1972). Stopwatches, unlike hand-operated counters, are rather expensive and, unfortunately, tend to disappear. However, they are necessary for measuring the latency of a behavior or behaviors of brief duration.

When you are using interval recording, particularly when the intervals are very short, glancing at the second hand on a watch or clock can be awkward and inaccurate. It is more convenient to have some sort of timer that will make a sound at the end of each interval. There are at least two ways to make yourself an inexpensive audible timer. One method, which has been described by Quilitch (1972), is a simple electronic device. The other option is to record a sound on an audiocassette at regular intervals and play the cassette on a portable tape recorder (Martin & Pear, 1978). Both of these devices can be used with an earphone so that the sound will not be heard by the individuals you are observing.

The most accurate way to use an audible timer is called *momentary interval recording* (Green & Alverson, 1978). This procedure involves recording whether the behavior you are measuring is occurring at the moment you hear the tone. There are other ways to use interval recording, but they tend to be less accurate than the momentary approach. Also, to improve accuracy, use intervals no more than 120 seconds long (Powell, Martindale, Kulp, Martindale, & Bauman, 1977).

It is occasionally very helpful to make tape recordings of behavior. Audio recordings are valuable if you are interested in verbal behavior, and can be made easily with a portable cassette recorder. Video recordings are even better, because you can record nonverbal and verbal behaviors, as well as the surroundings in which the behaviors occur. If your facility does not own video equipment, you may be able to borrow it from the public library or a nearby college or university. Tape recordings preserve events, making it possible to measure and/or analyze behavior at a later time (Sulzer & Mayer, 1972).

Exercises

6-15. Describe three approaches to recording behavior.
6-16. For what measurement approach(es) and/or dimensions of behavior would you use each of the recording tools listed below?
   a. Clock
   b. Stopwatch
   c. Forms
   d. Audible timer
   e. Wrist counter

Answers to Exercises

6-15. Continuous event recording, interval recording, time sampling.
6-16. a. Clock—all
   b. Stopwatch—latency, duration
   c. Form—all approaches, all dimensions
   d. Audible timer—interval recording
   e. Wrist counter—continuous event recording or time sampling of frequency

ISSUES IN MEASURING AND RECORDING BEHAVIOR

Who Measures?

At first glance this may appear to be a rather silly question. Who measures? Staff do, of course. That is often the only practical and reasonable answer to the question of who measures behavior, but it is not the only possible answer. Anyone in an individual's environment who is in a position to observe the behavior of interest may measure it. This might include relatives, bus drivers, sales clerks, or peers, to name a few. It is important not to assume that staff must be the ones who observe behavior (or implement programs), particularly since another answer to the question of who measures a person's behavior is that the person measures his or her own behavior. This is called self-monitoring or self-recording, which is discussed later in this section.

Reactivity

Several researchers have studied the effects of observation of behavior on the data collected. Often observers' recordings differ from what is really occurring because their recordings are *reactive*. One form of reactivity is *observer drift;* that is, over time observers tend to change the way they apply the definition of the behavior they observe (Kazdin, 1977). The reason agreement should be checked throughout a measurement period is to determine whether or not observer drift is occurring.

Another form of reactivity is *expectancy:* observers may record behavior as changing in the direction they expect, even though the change expected is not happening (Hersen & Barlow, 1976). This is *not* the same as faking data. People affected by expectancy record what they honestly believe they have seen. The possible presence of expectancy effects can be determined by periodically using someone who is not involved in the program to change a behavior as an observer. Ideally, that person should also not know what change in the behavior is desired, a condition that is often not possible to meet in applied settings. However, it is usually possible and always desirable to have someone who is not implementing a program measure its effects.

Another form of observer reactivity is the well-established reaction of observers to having interobserver agreement checked. In general, observers who know their agreement is being checked tend to show higher percentages of agreement than those who do not know. Unfortunately, the way to control for this reaction is to have observers believe that their agreement is either checked every time they observe or never checked (Kazdin, 1977).

Observers are not the only ones who may react to the observation process: it may also affect those being observed. How many times have you asked for help with a behavior problem only to have it disappear when help arrives? Little is known about how being observed affects behavior. There is generally agreement that there is a reaction to being observed. There is also agreement that the reaction disappears as people become used to the observation, or habituated, but no one knows how long this process occurs after observations are begun. The way to control for reactivity to being observed is to make observations as unpredictable and unobtrusive as possible (Wildman & Erickson, 1977). If observations are predictable (always occur at the same time), people are more likely to behave differently at the times that they know they are being observed. When observations are obtrusive, i.e., very obvious, people are more likely to be aware of them and therefore behave differently. That is why counters or other instruments that make loud noises, and other similarly obtrusive procedures should be avoided or made as unobtrusive as possible.

Observer Agreement

If the data you collect are to be meaningful, two different people should get the same results when they use the same definition and procedures to observe the same behavior. There are several ways to measure interobserver agreement.

When you are measuring frequency, the formula is:

$$\frac{\text{Smaller frequency}}{\text{Larger frequency}} \times 100 = \% \text{ Agreement}$$

For example:

Joe recorded 75 assembly units completed by the worker in 3 hours. Mary recorded 85 units completed during the same period.

$$\frac{75}{85} \times 100 = 88\% \text{ Agreement}$$

For duration it is (Gardner, 1977):

$$\frac{\text{Shorter duration}}{\text{Longer duration}} \times 100 = \% \text{ Agreement}$$

You can also check agreement of latency recordings with the duration formula. For example:

Observer 1 recorded total latency following a series of instructions as 63 seconds. Observer 2 recorded it as 54 seconds.

$$\frac{54}{63} \times 100 = 86\% \text{ Agreement}$$

A formula you can use for interval recording is:

$$\frac{\text{Total \# agreements}}{\text{Total \# agreements} + \text{total \# disagreements}} \times 100 = \% \text{ Agreement}$$

For example:

> Two observers used interval recording to determine the percentage of time an
> individual was on task. One observer recorded on-task behavior during 45 inter-
> vals of 50 observed. The second observer agreed with the first one during 43 of
> observer one's 45 on-task intervals and 2 of observer one's 5 off-task intervals.

$$\frac{43 + 2}{(43 + 2) + (2 + 3)} \times 100 = \frac{45}{50} \times 100 = .9 \times 100 = 90\% \text{ Agreement}$$

The most accurate way to measure agreement during interval recording is to
use an audible timer that both observers can hear at the same time (usually a
split earplug is used). Also, at least 50 intervals must be checked in order to
get a meaningful measure of agreement (Birkimer & Brown, 1979).

When you measure form, you typically check whether or not the observed behavior was of the correct form. When you measure intensity you
typically check whether or not the observed behavior was of the acceptable
intensity. Observer agreement for both these situations can be measured using
this formula:

$$\frac{\text{Total number agreements}}{\text{Total number agreements + total number disagreements}} \times 100 = \% \text{ Agreement}$$

The respectable standard for agreement is considered to be around 90%
(Gardner, 1977). If interobserver agreement is lower than 90%, you need to
look at possible reasons for failing to meet the standard. The most likely
reason is that the definition of the behavior being observed is not precise
enough (Sulzer & Mayer, 1972). Other possible causes of low agreement are
poorly designed data sheets or recording procedures, distractions during recording (Martin & Pear, 1978), or equipment failure. Observer agreement
should be checked when you first begin measuring a behavior, and then
checked regularly throughout the measurement period (Gardner, 1977).

Self-Monitoring

Having an individual record his or her own behavior can be useful for two
reasons. First, self-monitoring often results in positive behavior change (Nelson, 1977). This is called reactivity. Second, self-monitoring is an important
aspect of self-management. If your goal is to teach people to function independently, they must be able to manage their own behavior. Since people must
be able to monitor their behavior in order to manage it, self-monitoring is a
necessary prerequisite for self-management.

The problem with self-monitoring is that it is often not very accurate.
Some of the factors that may affect accuracy are whether the individual knows
accuracy is being checked, whether the individual is reinforced for accuracy,
whether desirable or undesirable behaviors are being monitored (undesirable

behaviors tend to be self-monitored less accurately), what the person is doing while he or she is self-monitoring, what type of training in self-monitoring has been given, and the nature of the self-monitoring procedure (Nelson, 1977).

There are ways to increase the accuracy of self-monitoring. One approach is to spot-check accuracy at randomly chosen times and provide rewards for accuracy and penalties for false data (Hundert & Bucher, 1978). Another approach is to teach people how to self-record accurately. In one recent study, a group of mentally retarded adolescents who were self-monitoring appropriate verbalizations in class were trained to improve their accuracy. They were shown videotapes of themselves in class and asked to record their behavior. Then they received additional practice in class with feedback on whether or not they were self-recording accurately. This procedure improved accuracy (Nelson, Lipinski, & Boykin, 1978). Other recommendations for promoting accuracy are: use simple data collection procedures that are compatible with the type of data being collected and, whenever feasible, have individuals record positive rather than negative behaviors (Mahoney, 1977).

Although it is possible to improve the accuracy of self-recording, the procedures used to do so will probably not affect reactivity. That is, accurate self-recording is just as likely to be reactive as inaccurate self-recording (Bornstein, Mungas, Quevillon, Kniivila, Miller, & Holombo, 1978). This is not necessarily a disadvantage because self-recording is often reactive in a positive direction.

Exercises

6-17.   Give three answers to the question of who measures.

6-18.   Describe three possible reactions to observation by the observer.

6-19.   What are some of the possible reactions to observation by the person being observed?

6-20.   Why is it important to check observer agreement?

6-21.   What are the advantages and disadvantages of self-monitoring?

6-22.   Observer A recorded 45 occurrences of a behavior during a time sample event recording, while Observer B recorded 40 occurrences. What is the interobserver agreement score for these two observers?

6-23.   The total duration of a man's time on task during a 2-hour work period was 63 minutes according to one observer and 72 minutes according to a second observer. What is their interobserver agreement score?

6-24.   Find the interobserver agreement score for these observations from an interval recording:

Observer 1	Y	Y	Y	Y	N	N	Y	Y	N	Y	Y	Y
Observer 2	Y	N	Y	Y	N	Y	Y	Y	N	Y	Y	Y

Y = behavior occurred, N = behavior did not occur

Answers to Exercises

6-17.   Staff, the person behaving, relatives, peers, etc.
6-18.   Drift, expectancy, increased agreement during known checking of agreement.
6-19.   Escape, more positive behavior, less positive behavior.
6-20.   To see if different observers get the same definition and procedures.
6-21.   Advantages—promotes independence, often positively reactive.
        Disadvantage—often inaccurate.

6-22. $\dfrac{40}{45} \times 100 = 89\%$

6-23. $\dfrac{63}{72} \times 100 = 87.5\%$

6-24. $\dfrac{8 + 2}{(8 + 2) + (1 + 1)} \times 100 = \dfrac{10}{12} \times 100 = .83 \times 100 = 83\%$

REPORTING BEHAVIOR

Drawing Graphs

A graph is simply a picture of data. A well-made graph provides a descriptive picture that summarizes the measurements you have obtained, a picture that is clear, simple, and explicit (Parsonson & Baer, 1978). Drawing useful graphs is easy if you follow a few simple guidelines. The most important guideline is to *always use a pencil*—it's a lot easier and neater to fix a mistake!

The specific steps in making a graph are:

1. **Draw the axes.**   These are the horizontal line at the bottom, usually called the x-axis, and the vertical line at the left, usually called the y-axis.

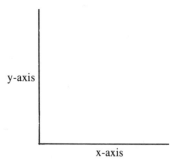

2. **Label the axes.**   When you graph behavioral data, the x-axis is usually time and the y-axis is usually the particular dimension of behavior you are measuring. Labels should be specific, not general. Don't use "time," use "days." Don't use "work rate," use "curtain rods assembled per hour."

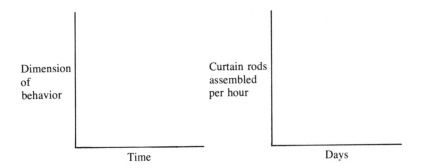

3. **Mark the scales.** Since the scales in this type of graph should be equal intervals, the easiest way to end up with an accurate graph is to use *graph paper*.
4. **Label the scales.** Use similar divisions on the two axes so that changes in behavior will not appear distorted (Parsonson & Baer, 1978).

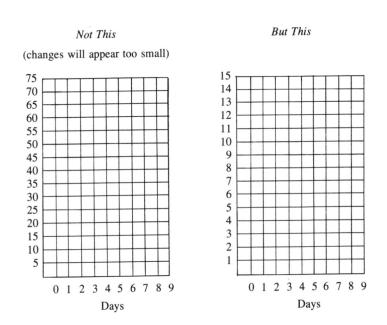

5. **Plot your data.** For each day (or each unit of the time period used) go to that day on the horizontal axis and then go up till you are directly to the right of the observed rate (or duration, etc.) on the vertical axis. Suppose you had these data:

Day	Rate of curtain rods assembled per hour
1	3.5
2	5.0
3	2.5
4	3.0
5	4.5
6	6.5
7	7.0
8	8.0
9	7.5
10	8.0

They would look like this when plotted on a graph:

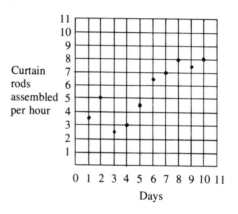

6. **Separate and label treatment conditions.** Suppose in our example that days 1–5 were baseline, with verbal praise for each assembly completed beginning on day 6. The labeled graph would look like this:

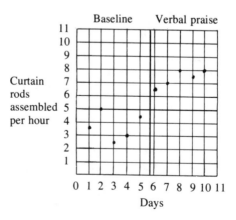

7. **Connect the data points within each treatment condition.**
8. **Title the graph.** The title should be a concise description of what you have graphed. For our example, the title could be:

Mary Smith's curtain rod assembly production

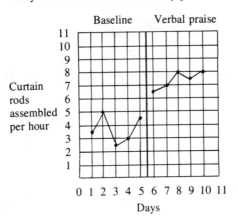

Interpreting Graphs

Once you have graphed your data, you will need to interpret them. The ultimate question is whether the behavior you have observed meets the criterion for success. An intermediate question is whether, if the criterion for success has not been met, programming has resulted in any change in behavior. Changes can occur in level, direction, or variability (Glass, Willson, & Gottman, 1975).

A *change in level,* in its simplest form, looks like this:

A *simple change in direction* could look like this:

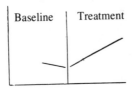

A *change in variability* might look like this:

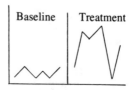

In addition, any of these changes may be delayed or temporary (Glass et al., 1975). A *delayed* change in level, for example, might look like this:

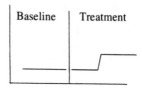

A *temporary* change in direction might appear in this form:

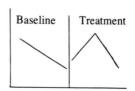

Be sure to look for all possible types of changes in your graphs. Although your programs may not always result in the changes you intend, sometimes you may find changes you didn't expect.

Exercises

Use graph paper to graph the data given below (6-25 through 6-27).

6-25.   A person interacted with peers for 45 minutes on day 1, for 39 minutes on day 2, for 52 minutes on day 3, for 40 minutes on day 4, and for 62 minutes on day 5. Graph the durations of the behavior for the five days.

6-26.   Calculate and graph the rates of correct greeting behavior for six days using the data provided below.

Day	Frequency	Total observation time	Rate
1	23	10 hr	
2	31	7 hr	
3	45	9 hr	
4	Absent	Absent	
5	42	9.5 hr	
6	44	10 hr	

6-27. Calculate and graph the percentages of compliance for 10 days using the data provided. *Note that treatment started on day 7.

Day	Number of requests	Number complied with	Percentage
1	12	6	
2	20	12	
3	15	12	
4	7	7	
5	9	7	
6	18	9	
*7	27	18	
8	16	14	
9	20	15	
10	12	9	

Tell what kind of change, if any, is shown in these graphs (6-28 through 6-31):

6-28.
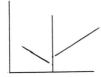

6-29.
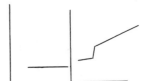

6-30.
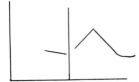

6-31.
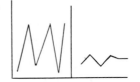

Answers to Exercises

6-25.
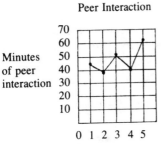

Peer Interaction

Minutes of peer interaction

70 60 50 40 30 20 10

0 1 2 3 4 5

Days

6-26.

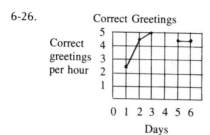

Correct Greetings

6-27.

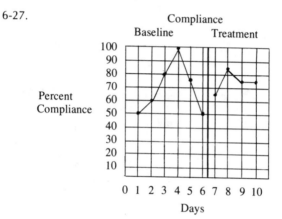

Compliance

6-28. Change in direction.
6-29. Delayed.
6-30. Temporary change in direction.
6-31. Change in variability.

CHOOSING MEASUREMENT, RECORDING, AND REPORTING PROCEDURES

This chapter has introduced you to the basic types of measuring, recording, and reporting used in behavioral assessment. However, in order to use these procedures effectively you also need a way to systematically decide which procedures to use in a particular situation. The guidelines given below are designed to provide you with a system for selecting appropriate assessment procedures. The Measurement Procedure Form, included on page 135, is designed to give you a quick and comprehensive description of your procedures once you have selected them.

Guidelines for Selecting Assessment Procedures

I. Take anecdotal records.
II. Operationally define the behavior being assessed.
III. Identify the relevant dimension of the behavior.

A. If how often the behavior occurs is relevant, the dimension is frequency.

B. If how long the behavior occurs is relevant, the dimension is duration.

C. If how long after the cue is presented the behavior occurs is relevant, the dimension is latency.

D. If how well the behavior conforms to a set standard is relevant, the dimension is form.

E. If how much of the behavior occurs is relevant, the dimension is intensity.

IV. Select the recording procedure.

A. Decide *when* to observe.

1. Choose continuous recording if behavior has a clear beginning and ending; choose interval recording if the behavior does not have a clear beginning and ending (Gardner, 1977) and if precise duration is not a major concern (Martin & Pear, 1978).

2. If using interval recording, choose the length of the interval—shorter intervals for shorter behaviors, longer intervals for longer, more continuous behaviors (Kazdin, 1975). In all cases choose intervals no less than 10 seconds and no more than 120 seconds in length.

3. Identify all times that the behavior may occur, on all days of the week. Then decide whether to observe during all those times or whether time sampling is necessary because of high frequency or long duration over long periods, or lack of observer time (Martin & Pear, 1978).

4. If using time sampling, choose the number of time samples per day or per week. Come as close as practical to having one sample for each period when the behavior may occur (Kazdin, 1975).

5. Choose the length of the time samples. Consider availability of observers, difficulty of recording procedures, and frequency of behavior (Kazdin, 1975).

6. Choose times for time samples that are representative of the periods of most interest. You may want to observe the behavior continuously for a day or two to identify those periods (Kazdin, 1975).

7. Decide the length of the baseline. Either pick a set length in advance or set a criterion for beginning the program. Never have less than three observation periods for baselines. For behaviors that are not extremely variable, roughly one or two weeks is usually an appropriate length for baseline.

      B.   Determine *who* will do the observing. Choose from individuals available in the settings selected (Martin & Pear, 1978).

      C.   Determine *where* observations are to occur by identifying all settings where the behavior occurs and choosing from those settings the ones in which it is practical to observe (Martin & Pear, 1978).

      D.   Identify and locate the tools needed to record observations (Martin & Pear, 1978).

          1.   Data sheet.

          2.   Other: Frequency—hand or wrist counter.
                    Duration or latency—stopwatch.
                    Interval recording—audible timer.

          3.   To preserve record, use audio or videotape.

      E.   Describe how to record.

  V.   Design a graph for the data.

  VI.   Design a procedure for assessing interobserver agreement.

  VII.   Check your procedures to see if anything more can be done to minimize the reactivity of observations. Ask yourself:

      A.   Are you assessing observer agreement throughout the measurement period to check for observer drift?

      B.   Is at least one of the observers not involved in implementing the behavior change program to control for expectancy?

      C.   Is it possible to avoid telling observers when their agreement is being checked?

      D.   Are the observations as unobtrusive and unpredictable as possible?

  VIII.   If self-monitoring is being used, check procedures to see that everything possible is being done to ensure that accurate recordings are made. Ask yourself:

      A.   Are positive behaviors being recorded?

      B.   Are accuracy checks to be done randomly?

      C.   Will the individual be rewarded for accuracy and penalized for inaccuracy?

  IX.   Arrange to train the observers to use the chosen procedures correctly. This includes accuracy training for self-monitoring.

  X.   Review all procedures and make sure that they are as simple as possible.

OTHER BEHAVIORAL ASSESSMENT PROCEDURES

There are a variety of behavioral assessment procedures in use in addition to those described in this chapter. Several of them are mentioned here so that you will be aware of their existence and can, if you wish, look for more information about them. If you are interested in a pattern of behaviors, such as how much time an individual spends interacting with others versus self-care versus being alone, you may want to observe using a *behavioral code*. Codes are appropriate for sampling several behaviors at the same time (Sulzer & Mayer, 1972). If you are interested in observing behaviors that are difficult to observe in natural settings or that naturally occur very seldom, you may want to use *role-playing*. In role-playing, the person is asked to behave as if he or she is in a particular situation (Gardner, 1977). This procedure is frequently used during the assessment and teaching of social skills. If you are interested in what individuals say to themselves, you may want to use *self-report* (Gardner, 1977). One use of self-report is to ask someone to say aloud what they ordinarily say to themselves while in a particular situation or performing a specific task.

There are many other behavioral assessment procedures available. The interested reader should consult one of the additional resources listed at the end of this chapter for further information.

SUGGESTED ACTIVITIES

The most important goal of this chapter is to teach you to select and use procedures for measuring, recording, and reporting behavior. So, take the Guidelines for Selecting Assessment Procedures and use them to select procedures for assessing a behavior of interest to you in your work. Then use the procedures you have selected to collect and record data and graph the results.

The more often you do this, the easier it will be to do it. Since you should be assessing behavior for every behavior change program you use, you'll get lots of practice!

ADDITIONAL RESOURCES

Cartwright, C. A., & Cartwright, G. P. *Developing observation skills.* New York: McGraw-Hill, 1974.

Cooper, J. O. *Measurement and analysis of behavioral techniques.* Columbus, Oh.: Charles E. Merrill, 1974.

Katzenberg, A. *How to draw graphs.* Kalamazoo, Mich.: Behaviordelia, 1970.

Korn, T. A., Ranney, W. C., Scheck, G. R., & Schober, D. K. *Behavior identification and analysis in rehabilitation facility services.* Menominee, Wisc.: Research & Training Center, 1976.

Meyers, C. H. *Handbook of basic graphs: A modern approach.* Belmont, Calif.: Dickenson, 1970.

Recommended procedure: *MDC behavior identification format.* Menominee, Wisc.: Materials Development Center, 1974.

AUDIOVISUAL MATERIALS

The following videotape can be rented or purchased from: Community Education & Technical Assistance Center, John F. Kennedy Child Development Center, Box C234, University of Colorado Health Sciences Center, Denver, CO 80262. (303)-394-8251

Rudrud, E., & Decker, D. *Observing and recording behavior*. Vermillion, S.D.: Center for the Developmentally Disabled, 1980. (Videotape)

REFERENCES

Birkimer, J. C., & Brown, J. H. Back to basics: Percentage agreement measures are adequate, but there are easier ways. *Journal of Applied Behavior Analysis*, 1979, *12*, 535–543.

Bornstein, P. H., Mungas, D. M., Quevillon, R. P., Kniivila, C. M., Miller, R. K., & Holombo, L. K. Self-monitoring training: Effects on reactivity and accuracy of self-observation. *Behavior Therapy*, 1978, *9*, 545–552.

Gardner, W. I. *Behavior modification in mental retardation*. Chicago: Aldine, 1971.

Gardner, W. I. *Learning and behavior characteristics of exceptional children and youth*. Boston: Allyn & Bacon, 1977.

Glass, G. V., Willson, V. L., & Gottman, J. M. *Design and analysis of time-series experiments*. Boulder, Colo.: Colorado Associated University Press, 1975.

Green, S. B., & Alverson, L. G. A comparison of indirect measures for long duration behaviors. *Journal of Applied Behavior Analysis*, 1978, *17*, 530.

Haywood, H. C., Filler, J. W., Jr., Shifman, M. A., & Chatelanat, G. Behavioral assessment in mental retardation. In P. McReynolds (Ed.), *Advances in psychological assessment* (Vol. 3). San Francisco: Jossey-Bass, 1975.

Hersen, M., & Barlow, D. H. *Single-case experimental designs: Strategies for studying behavior change*. New York: Pergamon, 1976.

Hundert, J., & Bucher, B. Pupils' self-scored arithmetic performance: A practical procedure for maintaining accuracy. *Journal of Applied Behavior Analysis*, 1978, *11*, 304.

Jones, R. R. *Intraindividual stability of behavioral observations: Implications for evaluating behavior modification treatment programs*. Paper presented at the meeting of the Western Psychological Association, Portland, Oregon, 1972.

Kazdin, A. E. *Behavior modification in applied settings*. Homewood, Ill.: Dorsey, 1975.

Kazdin, A. E. Artifact, bias, and complexity of assessment: The ABC's of reliability. *Journal of Applied Behavior Analysis*, 1977, *10*, 141–150.

Keefe, F. J., Kopel, S. A., & Gordon, S. B. *A practical guide to behavioral assessment*. New York: Springer, 1978.

Mahoney, M. J. Some applied issues in self-monitoring. In J. D. Cone & R. P. Hawkins (Eds.), *Behavioral assessment: New directions in clinical psychology*. New York: Brunner/Mazel, 1977.

Martin, G., & Pear, J. *Behavior modification: What it is and how to do it*. Englewood Cliffs, N.J.: Prentice-Hall, 1978.

Nelson, R. O. Methodological issues in assessment via self-monitoring. In J. D. Cone & R. P. Hawkins (Eds.), *Behavioral assessment: New directions in clinical psychology*. New York: Brunner/Mazel, 1977.

Nelson, R. O., Lipinski, D. P., & Boykin, R. A. The effects of self-recorders' training and the obtrusiveness of the self-recording device on the accuracy and reactivity of self-monitoring. *Behavior Therapy*, 1978, *9*, 200–208.

Panyan, M., Boozer, H., & Morris, N. Feedback to attendants as a reinforcer for applying operant techniques. *Journal of Applied Behavior Analysis*, 1970, *3*, 1–4.

Parsonson, B. S., & Baer, D. M. The analysis and presentation of graphic data. In T. R. Kratochwill (Ed.), *Single subject research: Strategies for evaluating change*. New York: Academic Press, 1978.

Powell, J., Martindale, B., Kulp, S., Martindale, A., & Bauman, R. Taking a closer look: Time sampling and measurement error. *Journal of Applied Behavior Analysis,* 1977, *10,* 325-332.

Quilitch, H. R. A portable, programmed, audible timer. *Journal of Applied Behavior Analysis,* 1972, *5,* 18.

Sulzer, B., & Mayer, G. R. *Behavior modification procedures for school personnel.* Hinsdale, Ill.: Dryden, 1972.

Warren, S. F., Rogers-Warren, A., & Baer, D. M. *Quality control in behavioral research: Two experimental analyses.* Paper presented at the 83rd Annual Convention of the American Psychological Association, Chicago, 1975.

Wildman, B. G., & Erickson, M. T. Methodological problems in behavioral observation. In J. D. Cone & R. P. Hawkins (Eds.), *Behavioral assessment: New directions in clinical psychology.* New York: Brunner/Mazel, 1977.

Anecdotal Record Form

Client _____ Observer _____ Date _____

Time	Antecedents	Behavior	Consequences	Location

Behavior Observation Form—Frequency

Behavior _____ Location _____
Client _____ Observer _____ Date _____

Time Observation Began	Time Observation Ended	Number of Occurrences	Rate

Behavior Observation Form—Duration

Behavior _____ Location _____
Client _____ Observer _____ Date _____

Time Observation Began	Time Observation Ended	Time Behavior Started	Time Behavior Stopped	Duration

Behavior Observation Form—Latency

Behavior _____ Location _____
Client _____ Observer _____ Date _____

Time Observation Began	Time Observation Ended	Time Cue Given	Time Behavior Started	Latency

Behavior Observation Form—Interval Recording

Behavior _____
Client _____ Observer _____ Date _____
Behavior observed _____ Location _____
Length of intervals = _____ seconds
Time started _____

Behavior Observation Form—Intensity

Behavior ___*Vocal Volume*___ Location ___*Group Home*___
Client _____ Observer _____ Date _____

Code: TL = too loud
TS = too soft
OK = acceptable
NT = not talking

Time	Code	Time	Code

Behavior Observation Form—Form

Behavior ___Ballpoint Pen Assembly___
Location ___Workshop_____

Client _____ Observer _____ Date _____

Time Observation Began	Time Observation Ended	Total # Pens Assembled	Total # Pens That Work

Measurement Procedure Form

1. Person to be observed _____
2. Operational definition of behavior to be observed _____
   _____
   _____
3. Dimension of behavior to be observed _____
4. When to observe
   a. days of week _____
   b. times of day _____
   c. dates _____
5. Who observes _____
6. Where to observe _____
7. Tools needed
   a. data sheet—attach to form
   b. other—include location of each item _____
      _____
      _____
8. How to record _____
   _____
9. Graph—attach to form
10. Procedures for assessing interobserver agreement _____
    _____
    _____
11. Procedures for minimizing reactivity _____
    _____
    _____
12. Procedures for training observers _____
    _____
    _____

Unit IV

Behavior Management
How Do We Get There?

Chapter 7

Behavior Principles

OBJECTIVES

To be able to:
1. Describe the key feature of the behavioral model presented in this chapter.
2. State the rationale for using a behavioral approach.
3. Define the A-B-C model of behavior.
4. Define discriminative stimulus.
5. Define S^D and S^Δ.
6. List and define the four ways that consequences can be used to alter behavior.

Chapter 1 introduced you to the first major aspect of our approach to habilitation programming: it is proactive. That is, we believe in a planned rather than a crisis-oriented approach. The second major aspect of our approach was covered in Chapters 4 and 5: it is individualized. We fit programs to people, not people to programs. Chapter 6 was devoted to the third major aspect of our approach: it is data based. We measure what we do and change it if it isn't working.

This chapter introduces you to the fourth major aspect of our approach: it is behavioral. We assume that most behavior is in large part dependent on factors in the environments in which it occurs (Kazdin, 1975). Furthermore, we are concerned primarily with those environmental factors that control behavior and that can be observed, measured, and altered. This way of looking at how a person behaves places the responsibility for behavior in the environment, not inside the person (Gardner, 1977). We cannot do much about genetic disorders, biochemical malfunctions, or birth defects. On the other hand, we can have an effect on what comes before a task (antecedents), what comes after a task (consequences), and task structure. Therefore, to change behavior you should change the environment in which it occurs. The use of a behavioral approach to habilitation does not allow us to blame program failures on "bad" or "sick" people. Instead, failures must be seen as the result of improperly designed or poorly implemented programs. This does not mean you are responsible for the success or failure of all your clients. You are responsible for program outcomes only when you are, in fact, in control of the environments in which those programs are implemented. If you are not in a position to alter environmental conditions, particularly consequences, you are not in a position to achieve program success.

RATIONALE

The reason we base our approach to habilitation programming on the behavioral model is very simple: it works.[1] To be more precise, it is the only model we are aware of that has led to considerable success in helping developmentally disabled people improve their adaptive living skills. This is not to say that the use of the behavioral model is a cure-all; it is not. Human behavior is so complex that no one can promise to be completely successful at changing it all the time. However, we are convinced that use of a behavioral approach will result in more success more of the time than use of any other approach.

Exercises

7-1. What is the key feature of the behavioral model and where does it place the responsibility for program success?
7-2. Why do we recommend using a behavioral approach to habilitation?

Answers to Exercises

7-1. The assumption that behavior is controlled by the environment. This assumption places the responsibility for successful programming with those in control of the environment, not with the client.
7-2. It works better more often than any other approach.

THE A-B-C MODEL OF BEHAVIOR

Overview

The A-B-C model of behavior provides us with a framework for deciding how behaviors can be modified (Sulzer-Azaroff & Mayer, 1977). It assumes that behavior is influenced by events in the environment. Events that occur immediately before a behavior are called antecedents, and events that immediately follow a behavior are called consequences. Behavior analysts are interested in examining the relationships between a behavior and its antecedents and consequences in order to identify those stimuli that may control

---

[1]Chapters 8, 9, 10, and 11 refer to specific examples of how the behavioral approach works.

behavior. Antecedents may set the occasion for the occurrence of a behavior, and consequences serve to either increase, maintain, or decrease a behavior.

We can easily see how this model works by examining our everyday environments. For example, when a traffic light turns red, most drivers will decrease speed and stop their cars. In this particular context, the red light has become an antecedent stimulus that precedes the response of stopping the car. There are many types of antecedents within our environments. However, not all antecedents control all behaviors. A red light may control the behavior of stopping a car, but a flashing yellow light will not necessarily control the same response. Also, a red light is a cue to stop their cars for most people, but not for an ambulance driver rushing a patient to the hospital. Antecedents can include the presence of a particular person or people, a sight, a sound, a smell, or a touch.

Positive consequences that follow a behavior can include events such as attention, praise, tokens, food, or water, or the removal of a negative event such as a loud noise. Negative consequences can be typically unfavorable events, such as reprimands, or the removal of something positive, such as attention.

Antecedents

Antecedents that consistently occur just before a behavior is reinforced may become signals that reinforcement is likely to occur. Other antecedents that consistently occur just before a behavior is not reinforced can become signals that reinforcement is not likely to occur (Kazdin, 1975). Both these types of antecedents are called *discriminative stimuli*. They allow the individual to discriminate between situations where the probability of reinforcement is high and those where it is not high.

We are concerned with two types of discriminative stimuli: an S^D, which signals that a behavior will likely be reinforced, and an S^Δ (read "S delta"), which signals that a response is not likely to be reinforced. For example, the telephone ringing can be an S^D since the probability of the response (answering and saying "hello") being reinforced (by subsequent conversation with the caller) is high. The phone not ringing is an S^Δ because the probability of the response being reinforced is low.

In a habilitation setting an S^D for a client's on-task behavior may be the presence of a particular trainer who consistently praises the client for being on-task. As a result, the client learns to be on-task in the presence of the trainer. The trainer has become an S^D for on-task behavior—because his or her presence indicates that reinforcement for on-task behavior is likely to occur. A trainer who neglects to praise the client for on-task behavior may easily become an S^Δ for that behavior. In the presence of such a trainer, the probability of reinforcement for on-task behavior is low. We encounter this frequently when staff express the concern: "The client will only work for Betty," or "She responds better to men." What we are really talking about are S^Ds and S^Δs.

Consequences

Consequences, the events that follow behavior, serve to increase, decrease, or maintain behavior (Powers & Osborne, 1976). In order to modify a behavior, consequences must be systematically delivered contingent upon the immediate occurrence of that behavior (Sulzer-Azaroff & Mayer, 1977). Behaviors will not be altered unless they are consistently followed by effective consequences. For example, one goal for Mary is to increase appropriate social interactions—specifically, saying "Good morning." The consequence for Mary's saying "Good morning" is an appropriate response such as, "Good morning, Mary." If after Mary says "Good morning" to a staff person she receives immediate recognition with a response, the probability of her behavior increasing is high. However, if the staff person ignores Mary's response, or does not respond until later on in the day, there will probably be little change in Mary's behavior.

There are two types of consequences—reinforcers and punishers. A *reinforcer* is any stimulus that, when presented contingent upon the occurrence of the behavior, increases the probability that the behavior will occur again (Powers & Osborne, 1976). A *punisher* is any stimulus that, when presented contingent upon the occurrence of the behavior, will decrease the probability of that behavior occurring again (Powers & Osborne, 1976). The most important thing about these definitions is that they are functional. Something is only a reinforcer for a particular individual if it strengthens that individual's behavior when presented contingently. If a given consequence does not strengthen a particular individual's behavior, it is not a reinforcer for that person. The definition of a punisher is also functional in that if a person's behavior is not decreased contingent upon presentation of the consequence, that consequence cannot be considered a punisher.

Reinforcers and punishers can either be presented or removed. Figure 7-1 shows the effects of the presentation or removal of the two types of conse-

	1	2
Increase responding	Present reinforcer	Remove punisher
Decrease responding	Present punisher	Remove reinforcer

Figure 7-1. Effects on behavior of the presentation or removal of the two types of consequences: reinforcers and punishers. (Adapted from Powers and Osborne, 1976.)

quences on behavior. In general, behavior can be increased by either present-ing a reinforcer or removing a punisher. Behavior can be decreased by either applying a punisher or removing a reinforcer.

Chapters 8, 9, and 10 present specific ways of using these principles to change behavior. We recommend that the overwhelming majority of all be-havior change programs be based on the presentation of positive conse-quences.

Exercises

7-3. What is an antecedent?
7-4. What is a consequence?
7-5. Define discriminative stimulus and describe the two types of discriminative stimuli presented in this chapter.
7-6. What are the two types of consequences?
7-7. How can consequences be used to increase or decrease behavior?

Answers to Exercises

7-3. An antecedent is something that occurs or is presented just before a be-havior is displayed.
7-4. A consequence is something that happens just after a behavior occurs.
7-5. Discriminative stimuli are antecedents that indicate how likely it is that a particular behavior will be reinforced. S^Ds indicate that the probability of reinforcement is high. S^Δs indicate that the probability of reinforcement is low.
7-6. Reinforcers and punishers.
7-7. To increase behavior, present reinforcers or remove punishers. To decrease behavior, present punishers or remove reinforcers.

SUGGESTED ACTIVITIES

1. Take a behavior of your own that you would like to change. Identify the antece-dents and consequences that appear to control that behavior.
2. What are the types of consequences typically available to clients served by your agency?
3. Given your answer to question 2, would you describe your agency as having a dominantly positive environment? If not, do you think the environment should be changed?

ADDITIONAL RESOURCES

Kazdin, A. *Behavior modification in applied settings*. Homewood, Ill.: Dorsey Press, 1980.

Martin, G., & Pear, J. *Behavior modification: What it is and how to do it*. Englewood Cliffs, N.J.: Prentice-Hall, 1978.

Reynolds, G. S. *A primer of operant conditioning*. Glenview, Ill.: Scott, Foresman, 1975.

Schwartz, B. *Psychology of learning and behavior*. New York: Norton, 1978.

Whaley, D., & Malott, R. *Elementary principles of behavior*. Englewood Cliffs, N.J.: Prentice-Hall, 1971.

REFERENCES

Gardner, W. *Learning and behavior characteristics of exceptional children and youth. A humanistic behavioral approach.* Boston: Allyn & Bacon, 1977.

Kazdin, A. E. *Behavior modification in applied settings.* Homewood, Ill.: Dorsey, 1975.

Powers, R., & Osborne, J. G. *Fundamentals of behavior.* St. Paul: West Publishing Co., 1976.

Sulzer, B., & Mayer, G. *Behavior modification procedures for school personnel.* Hinsdale, Ill.: Dryden, 1972.

Sulzer-Azaroff, B., & Mayer, G. *Applying behavior-analysis procedures with children and youth.* New York: Holt, Rinehart and Winston, 1977.

Chapter 8

Increasing Behaviors

OBJECTIVES

To be able to:

1. Define primary and secondary reinforcers.
2. State the functional relationship between primary and secondary reinforcers.
3. Describe four ways to select reinforcers.
4. Define the Premack Principle.
5. Define reinforcer sampling.
6. List the characteristics of behaviors under each of the following types of schedules of reinforcement: fixed interval, variable interval, fixed ratio, and variable ratio.
7. List advantages and disadvantages of using a continuous schedule of reinforcement.
8. List advantages and disadvantages of using intermittent schedules of reinforcement.
9. Give four guidelines for using reinforcers.
10. Describe the issues to consider when planning length and frequency of training sessions.

The proactive orientation has developed directly from observing difficulties in conceptualizing and implementing habilation programs for developmentally disabled clients. Generally, staff are better at identifying and knowing what they *don't* want clients to do than they are at identifying, developing, and carrying out programs for what they *do* want clients to do. The major goal and function of parents, educators, and human service workers is to teach new, functional, and appropriate behaviors. Behavioral programming has provided us with both the knowledge and the strategy to accomplish this task. The purpose of this chapter is to present the information needed to increase appropriate behaviors in clients.

ANTECEDENTS, BEHAVIOR, AND CONSEQUENCES

In Chapter 7, three critical elements were presented that need to be identified for each target behavior. These were:

1. *Antecedents,* or what comes before a behavior.
2. *Behavior.*
3. *Consequences,* or what comes after a behavior.

Antecedents

Antecedents or cues are those events in the environment that set the occasion for a behavior. All behaviors occur in the midst of a vast array of stimuli, and, although cues do not automatically "make" a response occur, they do communicate the likelihood of reinforcement of a certain behavior.

Exercises

8-1. The effects of cues on the behavior of clients can be readily seen. Observe clients in an educational or shop setting just prior to a regularly scheduled break. What do you notice?

8-2. When materials are laid out in order, Fred can initiate his work. If they are not laid out but are at the side of the room, Fred sits and stares.
   1. What is the S^D for work?
   2. By what method might you teach Fred to begin work all by himself?

Answers to Exercises

8-1. If there is a clock in the immediate vicinity you will no doubt observe many clients looking at the clock or you may notice decreases in the rates of attending to task, productivity, or on-task behavior. Similarly, you may observe increases in behaviors such as inattention, talking to neighbors, or leaving the work station. Thus, the clock serves as an antecedent or a cue that sets the occasion for break-related behaviors and negatively indicates work- or task-related behaviors. You may also notice that some clients only attend to a task when a staff person is in the immediate vicinity. The staff person in this case serves as a cue for on-task behavior.

8-2. 1. Clearly, having materials all laid out is an S^D for work for Fred.
   2. Slowly increasing the number of tools Fred must get on his own would be a way to gradually teach him to get his own materials.

By observing that certain behaviors are regularly preceded by certain cues, you can systematically alter cues in order to change behavior. In Exercise 8-1, what cues could you vary in order to decrease inattention and increase on-task behavior? What about the presence of the staff person cuing on-task behavior?

Variability in break time would likely decrease the amount of prebreak off-task behavior while simultaneously increasing the amount of on-task behavior. Also, variability in proximity of staff to clients can serve to alter on-task behavior. That is, if you slowly and systematically changed where the staff person stood, and only reinforced clients for time on task, it is likely that on-task behavior would increase regardless of where the staff person stood.

Consequences

Consequences are those things that follow a behavior that either increase or decrease the probability that the behavior will or will not occur again. Just as antecedents can be positive or negative, consequences can be either positive or negative. If you approach your supervisor with a problem and your supervisor says, "I don't have time for your troubles," that is a negative consequence and you are unlikely to bring similar problems to his or her attention. On the other hand, if your supervisor listens and expresses interest, the chances are that you would talk to him or her again. Positive consequences or positive reinforcement is one of the most powerful tools we have to increase behaviors. The use of positive reinforcement is also consistent with the proactive philosophy because it forces programming to focus on what we want the client *to do*.

Remember, a reinforcer is defined as *anything* that is presented *after* a behavior that *increases* the *probability* that the behavior will occur again. The principle of reinforcement has been verified by almost every major learning theorist, beginning with Guthrie (1935). It is important to critically examine this definition.

Defining Reinforcement The first important aspect of the definition of a reinforcer is that it is *anything* that increases or maintains a behavior. This means that reinforcement is highly individualized and based upon an individual's likes and dislikes. Literally, it is anything that works. You cannot decide automatically what will be reinforcing for another person. You must look at the individual's likes and dislikes.

Another key concept in the definition is that a reinforcer is something that comes *after* the behavior. This is different from a bribe that is promised, and sometimes delivered, before a behavior occurs. Powers and Osborne (1976) suggest that a bribe is more often involved when attempting to persuade a person to do something morally, ethically, or legally wrong. However defined, the distinction between a bribe and a reinforcer can seem confusing.

Exercise

8-3. Jenny's mother decides that Jenny should clean up her room before she does anything else that day. When approached, Jenny initially objects, but readily goes to work when her mother gives her a dollar. Two weeks later, Jenny again receives a dollar to "Go and clean your room."
   1. In two more weeks, what is likely to be Jenny's response to the command "Clean your room"?
   2. How else might the problem be approached?

Answers to Exercise

8-3. 1. If you think Jenny's response to the command "Go clean your room" would be "Sure, if I get my dollar," you're probably right. Remember, reinforcers always come *after* a behavior.

2. One solution to the initial problem is to ask Jenny to clean her room and allow her access to other favored activities (positive reinforcers) when she complies (and to be prepared for her objections and possible tantrum).

The next important part of the definition of a reinforcer is that it *increases* (or maintains) the probability a behavior will occur. This is a functional definition, which means that unless the behavior that you wish to increase or maintain increases or is maintained when you apply the consequence, then you are not using a positive reinforcer appropriate for that person. Therefore, the statement oftentimes heard, "I've tried positive reinforcement and it doesn't work," is meaningless. In order for anything to be a reinforcer it has to increase or maintain the behavior. The final aspect of the definition of a reinforcer is the word *probability*. Although we can usually be sure, we can't be completely certain of anything all the time when dealing with complex human beings.

Classes of Positive Reinforcement   There are two basic classes of positive reinforcement. The first class is *primary reinforcement*. Primary reinforcers are those things that are related to biological functioning. These include warmth, sex, comfort, and safety, although the most clinically useful and common primary reinforcers are those having to do with food and drink. Although specific types of reinforcers within this class may be learned (e.g., somebody may prefer liver and onions to cake or cookies), it is important to remember that, as a class, primary reinforcers enter the world along with the organism. Therefore, they are very powerful reinforcers and basic to maintenance of biological functioning. Primary reinforcement has been utilized to increase a variety of behaviors in clients. Meyerson, Kerr, and Michael (1967) taught a 9-year-old retarded girl to work utilizing edible reinforcers. Rudrud (1978) was able to reduce seizure rates in a severely retarded adult, and Whitman, Mercurio and Caponigri (1970) developed social responses in two severely retarded children utilizing edible reinforcers.

The other class of reinforcers is called *secondary reinforcers*. There are two important things to remember about secondary reinforcers: first, they are generalized from primary reinforcers and, second, their reinforcing properties are acquired via learning. Although we may come into the world needing and liking food, we have to learn to value the importance of reinforcers such as money, recreation, toys, or social interaction. When dealing with mentally retarded persons, very young children, or certain institutionalized populations, it is sometimes necessary and possible to teach them to enjoy certain reinforcing events. This is accomplished by repeatedly pairing something that the client does like—such as food—with something that has not yet been shown to be reinforcing to the person. By pairing verbal praise with cereal and slowly eliminating the cereal, we are able to teach someone how to work for a commonly available secondary reinforcer—verbal praise. The following example may help to illustrate this:

> Jim is a 37-year-old severely retarded man who spent the last 30 years in an institution. After 4 weeks in the day activity program, staff complained that, in the mornings and after scheduled breaks, Jim still did not return to his program area. Jim did not respond to verbal praise or reprimands from staff. One thing that he did enjoy was food. A backward chaining program, in which the last step in the chain (pick up work) was taught first, was developed to teach him to come to work on command. Edible reinforcers were repeatedly paired with verbal praise and pats on the back. After 5 days Jim was coming to his program area on command for verbal praise alone.

SELECTING REINFORCERS

One question often asked is, "How do you determine what are reinforcers for any individual?" There are four basic approaches. First, and simplest, is to ask the individual what he or she likes. From the responses, you can determine the most likely reinforcers for this person. Oftentimes, however, people have trouble specifying what they like. In these cases, the best solution is to utilize a reinforcer questionnaire that guides the person in specifying reinforcers. The reinforcer questionnaire included on pages 159-160 at the end of this chapter asks about favored events, objects, and activities. You can also utilize a list of possible reinforcers in determining positive reinforcers for the client. A sample list is provided immediately after the sample reinforcement questionnaire on pages 161-163.

The second method of finding out what is reinforcing to a person is to observe what that person does. In this case, you do not have to identify the reinforcer for the activity—only note that the person is engaged in doing something. This is based on the assumption that, because behavior is controlled by consequences, the person is receiving some sort of reinforcement for engaging in the behavior. This method can be very helpful when dealing with people who have either considerable difficulty expressing what they like or who don't seem to like much of anything. This procedure was developed by David Premack (1959) and it is known as the Premack Principle. What it suggests is that behavior can be divided into "high probability behaviors" and "low probability behaviors."

High probability behaviors are those things that a person, when left to his or her own devices, will do often. A low probability behavior is something that the person does not do very often. For example, when left alone, does a client attend to task or stare off into space? If the client stares off into space, then inattention is a high probability behavior and attention to task is a low probability behavior. Premack theorized that high probability behaviors could be utilized as reinforcers for low probability behaviors.

Exercise

8-4. Bill is a 45-year-old moderately retarded man who has barely adequate social skills that he seldom uses. He could get better with practice. In both the day activity program and residential setting, he usually keeps to himself. One of his identified needs is the need to increase the amount of time that he spends speaking to other staff and clients during social situations.
1. What is the major reinforcer for Bill?
2. How would you utilize the Premack Principle to increase social interaction?

Answers to Exercise

8-4. 1. Clearly, Bill's major reinforcer is time spent alone.
2. An example of the appropriate use of the Premack Principle would be that, after periods of social interaction, Bill would be able to spend time alone. Over time, the periods of "alone" time would be decreased and the periods of "social" time would be increased.

A third way to find out what is reinforcing to an individual is to utilize reinforcer sampling. In reinforcer sampling, individuals are given the opportunity to engage in a number of activities. They are then allowed to make choices about which reinforcers are preferred. This is a particularly effective method when working with mentally retarded clients. However, when introducing an individual to a reinforcer, we must present the reinforcer under optimal conditions. There is considerable evidence to suggest that, when a reinforcer is presented in a new situation, properties of that new situation can interfere with the effectiveness of the reinforcer (Sommer & Ayllon, 1956; Ferster & Skinner, 1957). For example, teaching a new task to a client would *not* be an optimal time to also introduce a new reinforcer.

In using reinforcers, we want to eliminate anything that may interfere with their effectiveness. One way to accomplish this is to have an individual client engage in the activity (intended reinforcer) prior to utilizing the activity or event as a reinforcer. By giving the client experience, we can then see if he or she will work to experience the reinforcer again. The reinforcer sampling rule is that, before using an event or a stimulus as a reinforcer, you should require sampling of the reinforcer in the situation in which it is to be used (Ayllon & Azrin, 1968). This is a particularly useful rule when an individual has no history of using the reinforcer and is therefore unfamiliar with it. Many times we make too many assumptions about clients. If a client has no history of fun with activities, satisfying personal relationships, or enjoyable experiences with certain foods, it is unlikely these events will be reinforcers until that history is established. For example:

Ayllon and Azrin (1968) describe the use of reinforcer sampling to increase the participation of institutionalized clients at a "social evening." The once-a-week evening included many activities such as bingo, dancing, and card playing. For the first 4 months of the program, all patients were required to participate for 5 minutes. Those who elected to stay paid one token, while all others were returned to the ward. The required attendance was then ended for 8 weeks but later was reinstated to demonstrate the effects of reinforcer sampling. Many more clients "bought" the reinforcer when sampling was required than when it was not. We can't expect mentally retarded clients to respond just because we think an event is reinforcing. Active sampling will provide the necessary familiarity.

The fourth and final way to determine reinforcers is by definition. Try something and see if it works. If you continually present an object, an event, or an activity after a desired behavior and the frequency of that behavior increases, then your consequence is reinforcing. In all cases, remember that reinforcement is defined by its effects on behavior. If the behavior does not change in the way that you want it to change, there is a high probability that your consequence is not a reinforcer for that particular individual.

Many programs utilize a token economy as a system of reinforcement for clients. Briefly, a token economy utilizes some sort of symbolic reinforcers (check marks, poker chips, play money) that are then exchanged for more tangible reinforcers (food, toys, activities). The specifics of a token program are well beyond the scope of this chapter. Indeed, there are several excellent books on the subject (Ayllon & Azrin, 1968; Kazdin, 1977). We would like to discourage most programs from utilizing token economies. This is not because they are ineffective (they work!) or artificial (they don't have to be!). It is because they are very, very difficult to run well. Most community-based programs simply do not have the expertise to effectively manage a token economy.

DELIVERY OF REINFORCERS

There are several factors that can influence the effectiveness of reinforcers. Some of the factors that are most important for you when working with clients include the schedule of reinforcement, the amount of reinforcement, and the timing of the reinforcement.

Schedules of Reinforcement

When a reinforcer is delivered is as important as what is delivered. The schedule of reinforcement refers to the relationship between the behavior emitted and the frequency of reinforcement. Ferster and Skinner (1957) delineated the major schedules of reinforcement. These have significant effects on the behavior emitted, and careful thought must be given to the schedule of reinforcement whenever a program designed to increase behavior is implemented (see Table 8-1).

Table 8-1.   Characteristics of behavior under different types of schedules of reinforcement[a]

Schedule	Characteristics of behavior
CRF	New behaviors acquired quickly, low frequency behaviors strengthened quickly.
	Extinguishes rapidly when reinforcment is withdrawn.
FR	Pause in responding after reinforcement delivered, then rapid increase in responding till next reinforcer delivered.
	Larger ratios result in larger pauses.
FI	Pause after reinforcement, increased rate as reinforcement time approaches.
	Behavior less consistent than under FR schedules.
VR	Responding consistently occurs at high rates.
	No pauses unless average ratio very long.
	Behavior very resistant to extinction.
VI	More rapid responding than under FI, but lower than under FR or VR schedules.
	Behavior very resistant to extinction.

[a]Source: Kazdin, A. E., 1975.

Continuous Reinforcement Schedule   In utilizing a continuous (CRF) schedule, every time a desired response is emitted, reinforcement is given. The relationship of behavior to reinforcement is 1:1. When teaching a new behavior, continuous reinforcement is the schedule of choice until the new behavior is established and success is achieved. Skill acquisition is quite rapid when a behavior is continuously reinforced.

Fixed Reinforcement Schedule   A fixed schedule is closely related to a continuous schedule, in that, for every set number of responses or period of time, reinforcement occurs. Whereas a continuous schedule has a behavior-to-reinforcement ratio of 1:1, that of a fixed schedule might be 5:1, 2:1, or 20:1. In any event it is fixed. Two variations on a fixed schedule are:

1. *Fixed ratio (FR)*—for every so many behaviors, a reinforcer will be delivered. For example, for every fifth widget Paul produces he receives 50¢. A continuous schedule is simply a fixed schedule that specifies a ratio of 1:1.
2. *Fixed interval (FI)*—whereas ratio refers to behavior, interval refers to time. For example, your pay check (it is hoped) is on a fixed interval schedule. Every month you get paid.

Variable Reinforcement Schedule   Variable reinforcement schedules differ from fixed schedules in that there is a changing pattern to the schedule.

Some, but not all, responses are reinforced. A variable schedule might be two responses before reinforcement, then six responses before reinforcement, then one response, then nine. In short, the client cannot depend on exactly *when* reinforcement is coming. Variable reinforcement has the advantage of serving to maintain a behavior for long periods of time without reinforcement. When a person has been learning a task on a continuous schedule, the behavior rapidly disappears when reinforcement is removed. How often would you flick a light switch if the light didn't come on? How long would you continue to work if you didn't receive a pay check this month? However, behaviors on variable schedules are more resistant to the loss of reinforcement. People playing a slot machine will persist in playing and losing money because they are reinforced on a variable schedule.

Most of the social behaviors exhibited by clients are on a variable schedule of reinforcement (Rosen, Clark, & Kivitz, 1977). This is both good news and bad news: good in the sense that appropriate behaviors will maintain, but bad because variably reinforced maladaptive behaviors are difficult to eliminate when necessary.

As suggested previously, when teaching a new behavior continuous reinforcement is best, but variable schedules are most effective to maintain a behavior. To change from continuous to variable reinforcement, gradually reduce the density or frequency of reinforcement. The main rule in reducing the reinforcer density is to *believe in the behavior*. That is, if performance begins to decrease, the density of reinforcement is being reduced too quickly.

Two different types of variable schedules are:

1. *Variable interval (VI)*—the amount of time between reinforcement is varied.
2. *Variable ratio (VR)*—the number of times the behavior must be emitted prior to reinforcement is varied.

Exercise

8-5. Can you identify the probable schedule of reinforcement for the following behaviors?
   1. Supervisor reprimands for client misbehavior.
   2. Clients buying candy or pop from a vending machine.
   3. A client who steals objects from other clients or staff.

Answers to Exercise

8-5. 1. If you said variable ratio or interval, you're right. From the description it would be difficult to know if the supervisor lets a behavior go for a period of time or catches behaviors every few times.
   2. Number 2 is a fixed or continuous schedule (if the machine is in good working order; if not, it is similar to the variable reinforcement of a slot machine).
   3. Number 3 is a variable ratio schedule: some behaviors get caught and some don't.

Guidelines for Using Reinforcers

Reinforce Consistently Regardless of how reinforcement is delivered, continuously or intermittently, it is necessary to reinforce consistently. When providing reinforcement for a new behavior it is necessary to specify which behavior is being reinforced. When you explicitly provide reinforcement for the occurrence of certain behaviors and do not provide reinforcement for other behaviors, your client will discriminate what behavior will result in reinforcement. Reinforced behaviors will increase. Additionally, other staff members need to be aware of what behaviors are to be reinforced so that consistent reinforcement can be provided.

If reinforcement is not provided consistently the behavior cannot be expected to increase, and at times superstitious behaviors may develop. Superstitious behavior results from the occasional chance pairing of a reinforcer with a response (Powers & Osborne, 1976). Superstitious behaviors are oftentimes seen in the gambling casinos—slot machine players will wear a lucky glove or hat because they were wearing those articles of clothing the last time they won. In order to reduce the occurrence of superstitious behaviors, reinforce consistently and specify the behavior(s) to be reinforced.

Reinforce Improvement When a client is asked to do something new or difficult he or she should be reinforced for progress. Do not wait for final accomplishment of the target behavior—reinforce small steps. For example, suppose a client is to learn a new task such as stapling pieces of paper together. Since the client has never stapled before he or she cannot know what is expected. The instructor could physically guide the client through each step of the procedure and then provide a reinforcer to the individual. For the next trial the instructor could provide physical assistance at the beginning of the procedure and let the client finish the last step independently. If the client succeeds in completing the stapling procedure he or she should be reinforced. The amount of assistance provided should be gradually decreased until the client can perform the task independently.

Pair Verbal Praise with Tangible Reinforcement Whenever tangible reinforcers are provided, pair verbal praise with the delivery of the reinforcer. Verbal praise is often not particularly effective. This is especially true with lower-functioning clients. However, by pairing verbal praise with the delivery of tangible reinforcers, verbal praise can acquire reinforcing properties. Verbal praise becomes a secondary or acquired reinforcer. Once verbal praise has acquired reinforcing properties, new behaviors can be taught and maintained by its use.

Reinforce Immediately When a client is learning a new task, success on that task should be reinforced immediately. Reinforcement is most effective when delivered immediately after the performance. The shorter the delay between the behavior and the reinforcement, the more effect the reinforcement will have on the behavior. When a client immediately goes to his or her work station and the instructor praises the client, going to the work station immediately will most likely increase. If the instructor waited until the end of the day to praise clients who immediately go to work, it is doubtful that going immediately to work would increase.

In addition to weakening the effect of the reinforcement, delay of reinforcement may result in the accidental reinforcement of an undesired behavior (Kazdin, 1975; Miller, 1978; Sloane, Buckholdt, Jenson, & Crandall, 1979). Coming to work, the director of a work activity center may observe a client being courteous and helpful to another client but may not say anything to the client. During the morning, the client has engaged in many undesirable behaviors. At lunch time the director sees the client and praises him for being very helpful. The behaviors that were reinforced were the undesirable behaviors rather than the helpfulness. Delivering reinforcement immediately prevents accidental reinforcement of undesirable behaviors.

PLANNING TRAINING SESSIONS

Little has been written about the structure of training sessions themselves. As pointed out in Chapter 1, many objectionable behaviors that clients exhibit are displayed in the course of social interactions, and thus much training is unstructured. However, for other behaviors, particularly skill development, training occurs at scheduled times. Whether training is scheduled or not, there are certain fundamental similarities between the two situations that must exist if client learning is to be maximized. Two important similarities, the number of trials and the duration of trials, can be easily translated into two questions we often hear: "How long should I train?" and "How often should I train?"

There are no simple answers to either of these questions. However, we do know that clients typically need many opportunities to sufficiently learn a skill. Whether it's appropriately approaching others or making a bed, too many programs intervene only when the behavior naturally occurs. If the client needs to learn to greet staff appropriately upon entering the building, and we only try to teach the skill when the client enters in the morning, how many learning trials per week does the client have? Of course, the answer is five.

This can be likened to learning how to play the guitar. Suppose you have decided that your real calling in life is to become a jazz guitarist. To accomplish this it is necessary to purchase a guitar, so you spend $1,000 on a brand new guitar. The next thing is lessons. Your instructor greets you, proceeds to take your shiny new guitar out of its case, and explains that the first chord to learn is the C chord. The instructor carefully positions your fingers and tells you to strum the guitar. Some sound resembling that of a broken clock spring bursts forth from the guitar. As you sheepishly grin the instructor says "good" and takes the guitar from your hands and announces that tomorrow you will practice again. How long will it take you to learn how to play the guitar? Probably you will not be able to master the guitar by being instructed this way. What is required is for you to have many repetitions until you can play one chord. Then you progress to the next.

Repetitions provide the opportunity for the client to emit a correct response. When the correct response occurs and positive reinforcement is provided, that response is strengthened and is more likely to occur again. The more times this correct behavior is reinforced the more likely it is that it will occur again; in short, the more learning trials the more likely the task will be learned. Although there is no set number of trials that is considered optimum, many instructors use a criterion of five consecutive correct trials before moving on to the next step or an 80% mastery of five or 10 trials. We prefer to use five consecutive correct trials before progressing to the next step.

Another parameter of the training session is the duration of the session: how long should we train? The duration of the training session is influenced by factors such as the mood of the learner, the schedule of reinforcement, the number of errors made during the session, the number of uncooperative responses, and so forth. In general, when training we suggest that the duration of the session not exceed 20–30 minutes. In fact, we generally prefer several intense sessions of brief duration during the day (e.g., 5–10 minutes).

Designing a Program

In the following exercise, identify the discriminative stimuli that you want to set the occasion for behavior. Which S^{D}s are presently associated with each behavior? Next, decide what you *want* the client *to* do. Avoid focusing on the excessive aspects of the client's behavior. Then select possible reinforcers. What schedule would you want to begin with: fixed interval or ratio?

Exercise

8-6. When Mary arrives at the activity center, she walks around shaking everyone's hand and says, "Good morning, how are you?" for the first 15 minutes. Whenever a visitor enters the work area, Mary immediately stops work, jumps up and shakes the person's hand, and interrupts whatever conversation is occurring.
1. What learning principle is maintaining Mary's behavior?
2. Can you identify the environmental antecedents?
3. How might you teach Mary to be more appropriate without suppressing her friendly nature?

Answers to Exercise

8-6. 1. If you believe that positive social reinforcement is maintaining Mary's behavior, chances are you are right.
2. The antecedents to her performance in the morning are probably the

time of day, the confusion when everyone is trying to get settled, and the approach of a staff member. How about when a visitor enters?

3. There are numerous programmatic options to increase Mary's in-seat behavior. One place to begin would be to socially reinforce her when she's in her seat.

SUGGESTED ACTIVITIES

1. Return to the list of agreed upon social behaviors that you developed in the activities section of Chapter 1. How many clients have goals for increasing these behaviors? For those who have a need, but aren't working on increasing one or more of the behaviors on the list, suggest a change in goals at the next staffing.

2. Observe clients as you work one day. Make a list of the primary and secondary reinforcers available for each of them.

3. Do all client intervention plans have notations about the schedule of reinforcement? Remember, schedules of reinforcement have an effect on the maintenance of behavior.

4. Describe how you would utilize the Premack Principle to:
   a. Increase the activity level of a client who only sat and watched TV.
   b. Increase time on task for a client who talked to his co-workers.

REFERENCES

Ayllon, T., & Azrin, N. *The token economy.* New York: Appleton-Century-Crofts, 1968.

Ferster, C. B., & Skinner, B. F. *Schedules of reinforcement.* New York: Appleton-Century-Crofts, 1957.

Guthrie, E. R. *The psychology of learning.* New York: Harper & Row, 1935.

Holland, J., & Skinner, B. F. *Analysis of behavior.* New York: McGraw-Hill, 1961.

Kazdin, A. E. *Behavior modification in applied settings.* Homewood, Ill.: Dorsey, 1975.

Kazdin, A. *The token economy: A review and evaluation.* New York: Plenum, 1977.

Meyerson, L., Kerr, N., & Michael, J. L. Behavior modification in rehabilitation. In S. W. Bijou & D. M. Baer (Eds.), *Child development: Readings in experimental analysis.* New York: Appleton-Century-Crofts, 1967.

Miller, L. M. *Behavior management: The new science of managing people at work.* New York: Wiley, 1978.

Powers, R. B., & Osborne, J. G. *Fundamentals of behavior.* New York: West Publishing Co., 1976.

Premack, D. Toward empirical behavior laws: 1. Positive reinforcement. *Psychological Review,* 1959, *66,* 219–233.

Rosen, M., Clark, G., & Kivitz, M. *Habilitation of the handicapped.* Baltimore: University Park Press, 1977.

Rudrud, E. *Eight to twelve Hertz occipital EEG training with moderately and severely retarded epileptic individuals.* Unpublished doctoral dissertation, Utah State University, Logan, 1978.

Sloane, H. N., Buckholdt, D. R., Jenson, W. R., & Crandall, J. A. *Structured teaching: A design for classroom management and instruction.* Champaign, Ill.: Research Press, 1979.

Sommer, R., & Ayllon T. Perception and monetary reinforcement: The effects of rewards in the tactile modality. *Journal of Psychology,* 1956, *42,* 137–141.

Whitman, T., Mercurio, J. R., & Caponigri, V. Development of social responses in two severely retarded children. *Journal of Applied Behavior Analysis,* 1970, *3,* 133–138.

Reinforcer Questionnaire

NAME _____
DATE _____
PROGRAM _____

1. My favorite person is _____
   Things I like to do with him or her are _____
   _____

2. The best reward anybody can give me is _____
   _____

3. My favorite job at work (or home) is _____
4. If I had 10 dollars, I'd _____
   _____

5. My favorite relative in _____ is _____
   (hometown)
6. For a job, I want to be _____
7. The person I dislike most is _____
   Why? _____
8. Two things I like to do best are _____
   _____

9. My favorite staff person is _____
10. When I do something well, the staff _____
    _____

11. I feel terrific when _____
    _____

12. The way I get money is _____
    _____

13. When I have money, I like to _____
    _____

14. When I'm in trouble, I _____
    _____

15. Something I really want is _____
    _____

16. If I had a chance, I sure would like to _____
    _____

17. The person I like most to reward me is _____
    How? _____
18. I really hate to _____
    _____

19. The thing I like to do best with my mother (father) is _____
    _____

20. The thing I do that bothers staff the most is _____
    _____

21. The weekend activity or entertainment I enjoy most is _____
    _____

22. If I did better work, I wish my instructors would _____
    _____
    _____

(continued)

Reinforcer Questionnaire (continued)

23. The kind of punishment I hate most is _____
_____

24. My favorite food is _____
_____

25. It sure makes me mad when I can't _____
_____

26. My favorite sport is _____
_____

27. My favorite brother or sister in _____ is _____
(hometown)

28. The thing I like to do most is _____
_____

29. The only person I will take advice from is _____
30. My two favorite TV programs are _____
Other activites I enjoy:

_____
_____
_____
_____
_____
_____
_____
_____

Possible Reinforcers

Please note: Many of the possible reinforcers listed here are not age-appropriate for adults. However, they may be the only ones your clients will respond to at first. Also, many of these reinforcers have been used successfully with children. Be sure you always pair an age-inappropriate reinforcer with an age-appropriate consequence that you want to become reinforcing to your clients. In other words, teach your clients to respond to age-appropriate reinforcers.

Food

Hot chocolate	Milk	Cookies
Popcorn	Coffee	Donut
Peanuts	Juices	Sweet roll
Animal crackers	Raisins	Fruit
Cereal	Tea	

A Positive Approach

Patting shoulder	Eating with	Helping put on coat
Straightening clothes	Standing alongside	Talking with
Shaking hands	Touching arm	Sitting near
Patting cheek	Touching hand	Walking alongside
Leaning over	Squeezing hand	

Expressions of Approval

Looking	Signaling O.K.	Raising eyebrows
Winking	Shrugging shoulders	Slowly closing eyes
Grinning	Cheering	Chuckling
Opening eyes	Smiling	Thumbs up
Laughing	Nodding	Whistling

Words and Written Symbols of Approval

Bravo	Good	Nicely done
Fine	Very good	Complete
Neat	Passing	A, B
O.K.	X	Enjoyable
★	100%	Excellent
Well done	Great	Outstanding
Wow	A-1	Colored pencil markings
Perceptive	Good work	Superior
Correct	+	Congratulations
Improvements	Satisfactory	

Things

Tokens	Pencil sharpeners	Elastic bands
Paint brushes	Paycheck	Paper clips
Book covers	Money	Colored paper

(continued)

Things (*continued*)

Paints	Pencil holder	Flowers
Records	Stationery	Chalk
Flash cards	Compasses	Clay
Surprise packages	Calendars	Perfume
Bookmarkers	Pictures	Radio
Pencils with names	Musical instruments	Magazines
Seasonal cards	Drawing paper	Newspaper

Individual Activities and Privileges

Free time
Leading groups
Representing group in activities
Putting away materials
Running errands
Choosing activities
Show and Tell (any level)
Dusting, erasing, cleaning, arranging chairs, etc.

Helping others—drinking, lavatory, cleaning, etc.
Answering questions
Outside supervising—patrols, directing parking, ushering, etc.
Assisting teacher to teach
Leading discussions
Displaying work

Social

Movies
Presenting skits
Playing records
Preparing for holidays
Playing games
Field trips
Planning daily schedules
Dancing

Going to museum, fire station, courthouse, picnics, etc.
Participating in group organizations (music, speech, athletics, social clubs)
Parties
Talent shows (jokes, reading, music, etc.)

Playthings

Cartoons	Puzzles	Jumping beans
Flashlight	Combs	Masks
Rings	Comics	Straw hats
Athletic equipment	Jump ropes	Banks
Tape recorders	Balloons	Address books
Badges	Commercial games	Fans
Pins	Yo-Yo's	Play Dough
Ribbons	Stamps	Whistles
Balls	Bean bags	

Reinforcers That May Be Used in the Home

Money
Verbal praise
Pat on back
Extra TV time
Extra time before going to bed
Watch more TV shows
New clothes

Have friend over for dinner
Choose TV program
Play game with friends, staff
Have a picnic
Making something in the kitchen
Have breakfast in bed
Wrap Christmas gifts

(*continued*)

Reinforcers That May Be Used in the Home (continued)

Entertain friends
Extra helping at dinner
Choose a particular food
Go to a movie
Go to the zoo
Records
Swimming
Parties
Charting
Friend to spend the night

Choose gift for friend
Fewer chores
Sleep later on weekends
Go on errands
Go out to a special restaurant
Take pictures of friends
Not have to wash clothes for a week
Not have to iron own clothes for a week
Start fire in fireplace
Put things on wall

Reinforcers That May Be Used in the Workshop

Supervisor's attention
Charting production rate
Time alone with another client
Pop
Coffee
Tea
Rolls during coffee break
Time alone with staff member

Going out to lunch
Working on special task
Building own project
Learning to operate new
    tool/machinery
Variation in tasks
Reading newspaper

Chapter 9

Teaching New Behaviors

OBJECTIVES

To be able to:
1. Define task analysis.
2. Define shaping.
3. List four types of prompts.
4. Define fading and indicate reasons why it is necessary.
5. Define imitation and indicate how it may be utilized effectively.
6. Define forward and backward chaining and provide examples.
7. Construct a forward chaining program.
8. Construct a backward chaining program.

Chapter 8 discussed ways to program for the increase of behaviors a person can already do. This chapter is devoted to techniques for teaching new behaviors, that is, skills a person has not already learned. As you go through this chapter, it is important to remember that programs designed to teach new behaviors must use the principles and procedures covered in *both* Chapters 8 and 9. This is because the best teaching program in the world will not succeed unless the skills taught are reinforced and practiced.

TASK ANALYSIS

Virtually every behavior, task, and educational objective is comprised of specific behavioral components or skills. A task analysis breaks a task down into specific components. When teaching new behaviors it is essential for each component of the behavior to be taught and mastered. The purpose of a task analysis is to provide a description of the specific skills the learner must acquire in order to learn the behavior. A task analysis provides for a detailed assessment of the learner's entry level abilities and specific prescriptive information about how to accomplish the goal or objective of the program. In other words, the task analysis helps pinpoint the current functioning level of the client and provides a basis for sequential instruction.

Guidelines

Training involves two basic objectives: teaching the client how to perform specific task-relevant behaviors and teaching the client when to perform those behaviors. Training can be conceptualized as building a chain of specific responses or behaviors. For example, the task of washing one's hands is not one behavior; rather, it can be viewed as many separate behaviors, as shown in Figure 9-1. Teaching hand washing can be thought of as building a chain of responses. Each response in the chain is cued by a different discriminative stimulus. When the client is given the verbal instruction to "please wash your hands," that serves as a discriminative stimulus and cues the response of pushing up his or her sleeves. Each response of the task analysis also serves as a discriminative stimulus for the next response. Pushing up sleeves is the cue for turning on the faucets, because the client must push up his or her sleeves before he or she turns the faucets on.

In developing a task analysis, the scope of the main task should be limited. It is not feasible to develop a task analysis for good personal hygiene. Instead, each component should be broken down into a specific task analysis, such as showering, hand washing, brushing teeth, shampooing hair, using deodorant, shaving, setting hair, and so on. Additionally, any task can be performed in a variety of ways. Oftentimes there is no right or wrong way to perform a task. In general, the design of the task analysis should be balanced between making the task easier to train and maximizing completion of the task. In designing the task, four basic rules that should be utilized are:

1. Minimize the number of different discriminations a client needs to make. For example, in a complex assembly task, place component parts in bins that are ordered in the way the parts are assembled rather than having the client sort as well as assemble.
2. Use a unique set of stimuli to cue each response. For example, don't use the cue "put the plates on the table" if there are several types of plates in the cupboard. Appropriate cues focus on what is unique about the stimulus.
3. When one operation is both repeated several times and performed in a slightly modified form, teach the general case before teaching the exceptions. For example, in bowling the general case is that for each turn you roll the ball twice. However, there is an exception when you get a strike (all 10 pins down with the first ball).
4. Maximize the use of concepts and operations already in the client's

repertoire. For example, if the client already knows *big* and *little*, don't use *large* and *small* as cues in teaching something else.

Development of the Task Analysis

After the scope of the task has been limited, the next step is to develop the task analysis. The subtasks must be written in observable terms and should focus on what the learner will do. These become the steps of the task analysis and should identify observable behaviors that are to be performed by the worker.

There are several methods that can be utilized when developing a task analysis (Moyer & Dardig, 1978). These include:

1. *Watch a master perform*—This requires good observational skills. The basic procedure is to watch a person who is proficient in the performance of the task complete it. As each step is completed, write down in correct order all steps performed. This is particularly useful in the development of task analyses for skills such as tying a shoe or sawing.

2. *Perform the task yourself*—When an expert is not available to demonstrate the task the instructor should perform it. This is a very useful technique but it may become difficult to stop the task and write down all of the steps. It is helpful to use a tape recorder to verbalize each step as it is performed and transcribe the steps later.

3. *Work backward through the task*—Oftentimes when constructing a task analysis, staff are too familiar with the task and as a result omit certain key steps when writing the analysis. One procedure that may help to reduce these oversights is to work backward through the task. One starts with the terminal objective and writes down those behaviors that immediately precede the terminal behavior. Each behavior is treated as the main goal and the process is repeated until you arrive at the entry level skill.

4. *Brainstorming*—Brainstorming is extremely useful for analyzing complex tasks that do not conform to a strict temporal sequence: for example, making change for a dollar or purchasing a jacket. Several staff members should get together and write down all subtasks involved in a goal and then arrange the subtasks in a logical order.

5. *Break down complex goals*—This method of task analysis is used most successfully with goals from the affective domain (Moyer & Dardig, 1978). The purpose of this type of task analysis is not to develop a list of sequential subgoals but to identify the specific behaviors that signal attainment of the goal. The steps included are:
   a. Write the goal.
   b. List observable behaviors that the client would exhibit showing attainment of the goal.

c. Discard those behaviors that should not be listed and clarify the remaining behaviors.
d. Describe how frequently and how well the behavior must be performed for each goal.
e. Test the list of behaviors to see if they represent comprehensive attainment of the goal.

Review of Task Analysis

After the task analysis has been completed it should be reviewed to determine whether or not it conforms to certain basic requirements. A checklist of the requirements includes:

1. Are all of the steps of the task analysis stated in observable and measurable terms?
2. Are any critical steps omitted? Can the learner perform the task after mastering the steps?
3. Are all steps or subtasks relevant to the goal?
4. Are any subtasks unnecessary?
5. Are the subtasks arranged in a sequential and logical order?

It is also necessary to test the task analysis in trial training sessions. The instructor should attempt to train the specific subtasks and keep accurate notes regarding a client's progress. Areas of difficulty can be noted, and if the client continues to have difficulty with one particular subtask, this would suggest that the one subtask may be too complex. If it is too complex it should be broken down into smaller steps. One of our biases is that if the learner is not progressing it's the fault of the program, not the fault of the learner. Go back, review the program, review the troubleshooting guide in Chapter 12, and begin again.

Oftentimes using a task analysis in a trial session is less efficient than testing it on another staff member. Using another staff member allows the instructor to get verbal feedback from difficulties the learner encounters. When using this procedure it is necessary for the other staff member not to assume what is implied in the subtask but to perform the subtask as specified in the task analysis. For example, in sweeping the floor the subtask may be written that the learner should "grasp the broom." A staff member would most likely pick up the broom correctly; however, a client who has not used a broom previously may grasp the broom upside down, sideways, or with only one hand. Each behavior must be accurately described so that the instructor knows exactly what is required.

Task Analysis Sheet

After the task analysis has been constructed it is best to make a data sheet. A basic data sheet is shown in Figure 9-1. This task analysis data sheet contains pertinent information regarding the client, potential reinforcers, materials needed, and a task statement to cue the learner. Each substep of the program is written in sequential order (in this example, hand washing is comprised of 15 sequential steps). To the right of each step are several columns. Each column represents a training session and is dated.

In the top right-hand corner of the task analysis data sheet is a scoring summary. This allows the instructor to rate how much assistance the client required in completing the steps trained during the session. A score of 3 indicates that the client performed the step independently. A score of 2 indicates that the client required verbal assistance, and a score of 1 indicates that the instructor either modeled the correct response or used gestures to communicate the correct response. A score of 0 indicates that the client either required physical assistance or made no response.

When utilizing this data sheet each training session should be represented in one column. During the training session the instructor should provide many trials on the step being learned. When the client performs that step independently, training may proceed to the next step.

At the end of the training session the instructor should take the client through the entire task analysis, scoring each step as to how much assistance the client required. The bottom of each column lists the number of steps scored as 3, or how may steps the client performed independently. These data can easily be charted on graph paper.

Exercise
9-1. Define task analysis and list five procedures that can be utilized to develop a task analysis.

Answer to Exercise
9-1. A task analysis breaks down a task into its specific components or subskills. The task analysis can be developed by utilizing the following methodologies:
1. Watch a master perform.
2. Perform the task yourself.
3. Work backward through the task.
4. Brainstorm.
5. Break down complex goals.

SHAPING

When a behavior does not exist in the learner's repertoire the instructor cannot provide reinforcement for the occurrence of that behavior. Then a shaping procedure must be used to create the behavior. Shaping refers to a procedure in which better and better approximations of the behavior are reinforced. Successive approximations of the desired behavior are reinforced until the objective is reached.

Task Analysis of Hand Washing

Program _____ Hand washing _____

Client _____

Instructor _____

Reinforcers _____

Materials _Towels, soap_____

Task Statement "_____, please wash your hands."

Dates:

1. Pushes up sleeves									
2. Turns up faucets									
3. Adjusts water temp. & pressure									
4. Wets hands									
5. Picks up soap									
6. Lathers soap									
7. Puts soap down									
8. Washes palms									
9. Washes between fingers									
10. Washes back of hands									
11. Rinses off soap									
12. Turns off faucet									
13. Picks up towel									
14. Dries hands									
15. Disposes of towel properly									
16.									
17.									
18.									
19.									
20.									
21.									
22.									
23.									
24.									
25.									

Number of steps scored 3:									

Figure 9-1. Sample task analysis data sheet for hand washing.

One common use of shaping is to teach new work behaviors. For instance, a client was to learn the task of sanding a piece of wood. To begin, the sandpaper and wood were presented and the trainer asked the client to sand the wood. The client was reinforced for successive approximations of the goal behavior to sand the wood. Reinforcement was delivered first for picking up the sandpaper, then for placing the sandpaper on the wood, then for making a sanding motion, then for additional sanding motions, and finally for longer and longer periods of time sanding. The client was differentially reinforced for sanding (i.e., reinforcement was presented when the client sanded and was not presented when the client was not sanding).

Another example of shaping was used by us to teach a client to "go to work." The client was a 37-year-old male who was profoundly retarded. The problem was that during break time the client would sit outside of the building. When it was time to return to work the client refused, and it usually required three or four staff to carry him back to the activities center. A shaping procedure was utilized to solve this problem. The client was at his table sitting in his chair. His work was placed in front of him and he was given the instruction, "It's time to go to work." When the client picked up his work he received social and edible reinforcers. After several correct trials the client and his chair were moved away from the table. When the verbal command was given the client was required to scoot his chair up to the table and pick up his work in order to receive reinforcement. After several successful trials the client stood next to his chair. In order to be reinforced the client had to sit in his chair, scoot up to the table, and pick up his work. Again after several successful trials the client stood behind his chair. The reinforced response consisted of moving to the front of this chair, sitting down, scooting up to the table, and picking up his work. The last trials consisted of the client standing further and further from his chair until he was outside the building, then walking to the chair, sitting down, scooting his chair to the table, and picking up his work. The entire shaping procedure required 15–20 minutes. The client mastered the task of coming to work and 6-month follow-up data indicated that the client came to work whenever he was requested.

PROMPTING AND FADING

Prompts are methods of teaching new behaviors. There are several types of prompts, including physical, gestural, verbal, and imitative. Clients may learn a behavior more quickly if guided in a manner that ensures few errors. Prompts are used to facilitate the acquisition of the new behavior by reducing the number of errors so that the behavior can occur correctly and be reinforced.

Physical prompts refer to situations in which the instructor physically assists the learner in performing the task. In teaching a client to sweep the floor the instructor may stand behind the client and place his or her hands over the client's hands while the client is holding the broom. It should be noted that the instructor is not doing the task for the client. Rather, guidance is being provided and the physical prompt will be faded so that the client performs the entire task independently.

A gestural prompt is one in which the instructor makes a gesture to indicate the correct response. In sweeping, the instructor may point to the broom or point to the floor. Gestural prompts are often used to indicate the correct response when several choices are presented. For example, an instructor who is teaching a client to choose a cup when presented with three additional objects may say "Sally, pick up the cup," and at the same time point to the cup.

Verbal prompts refer to verbal instruction. In sweeping the floor the instructor may tell the client to pick up the broom, how to hold the broom, how to make a sweeping motion, and so on.

Imitative prompts are prompts in which the instructor demonstrates the correct response. In sweeping the floor the instructor could hold the broom and make a sweeping motion to demonstrate the correct response.

Regardless of which type of prompt is used, it should be remembered that the prompt is used to exert temporary control over the behavior. Eventually the learner must perform the behavior without the prompt. This is done by fading. Fading refers to the gradual removal of prompts. As the desired behavior becomes strengthened the prompts should be removed. Generally speaking, prompts are faded by first removing those that require the most staff assistance (physical prompt) and then removing those that require less staff assistance (instructive prompt).

Prompts should not be maintained for an excessive length of time because the learner may depend upon them too much. Gardner (1977) stated that the general rule is to remove the prompts as quickly as possible without allowing the behavior to abruptly stop.

The instructor must also be aware of the individual differences among handicapped individuals. Each individual acquires new behaviors at different rates, will require different types of prompts, will need prompts for varying lengths of time, and will require different ways of fading the prompts.

IMITATION (MODELING)

Imitation, or modeling, is another useful technique in teaching new behaviors. As noted by Sloane, Buckholdt, Jenson, and Crandall (1979), children who have been reinforced for imitating others in the past are likely to imitate new behaviors when requested. This is particularly true if they have seen someone else being reinforced for performing that particular behavior.

Imitation is a very important way in which people learn many new behaviors. A step-by-step procedure for establishing or improving imitative skills is provided by Striefel (1977) in *Teaching a Child to Imitate*. Imitation can be used to teach a variety of behaviors and has particular utility in teaching on-task and attentive behaviors in group situations. By reinforcing those individuals who are on task, on-task behavior is increased and/or maintained. Those individuals who were not on task do not receive reinforcement. However, they have seen other individuals receive reinforcement and are thus provided models to imitate.

CHAINING

Most goals and objectives of the Individualized Program Plan represent complex behaviors. The goals are usually comprised of a number of discrete behaviors that the individual may or may not exhibit. For those discrete behaviors that the individual does not exhibit, a shaping procedure is utilized. When the discrete behaviors are combined to form complex behaviors, we refer to the process as chaining. For example, a client may know individually how to sit in a chair, work on a task, begin work, work extended periods without reinforcement, and put his or her work away. These are all behaviors that may be combined to form the complex chain called "work."

Gagne (1970) identified five conditions that are essential for effective learning of complex sequences of behavior. These include:

1. The individual components must be in the person's repertoire.
2. The individual components must occur sequentially in the correct order.
3. The individual components must be performed in close time succession.
4. The sequence of responses must be repeated to ensure that the rough spots are eliminated and that forgetting is prevented.
5. The sequence of behaviors must be followed immediately by reinforcing consequences.

Forward and Backward Chaining

When teaching the behavioral components of complex behavior there are two approaches that may be utilized—forward and backward chaining. Both forward and backward chaining require that the complex behavior be broken down into sequential components. The hand washing task analysis shown in Figure 9-1 can be taught by using either a forward or backward chaining procedure.

In forward chaining the instructor would begin by teaching the first step of the task analysis, removing jewelry and pushing up sleeves, and add sequential steps as each step is mastered. Reinforcement is provided for increasingly longer sequences of behavior. The entire sequence of the behavior is maintained by the final reinforcement provided by the instructor.

Backward chaining refers to a procedure in which the final step of the task analysis is taught first and the other preceding segments of the behavior are gradually added. In the hand washing task analysis the final step is hanging up the towel. In a backward chaining procedure, this behavior is taught first and, as the learner hangs up the towel, reinforcement is delivered. Once this behavior occurs when required, the preceding step (drying hands) is taught. In backward chaining the reinforcer is always delivered upon the completion of the last step of the behavioral chain. Thus, reinforcement serves to strengthen the entire sequence from beginning to end. Reinforcement is paired with the completion of a task.

There are no set guidelines as to when to use forward or backward chaining procedures. Which one to use depends on the task (tasks like swimming can't be backward chained), the learner, and the trainer (use procedures you have had success with in the past).

SUMMARY

In teaching new behaviors it is essential to have a good working knowledge of the principles of reinforcement. Furthermore, teaching new behaviors is often facilitated when the task is broken down into its sequential components. The use of a task analysis facilitates this process. Once the behavioral components have been identified it is necessary to determine whether or not the client exhibits the behavior. If the client cannot perform the behavior, then shaping, modeling, and/or prompting techniques need to be utilized.

When teaching the components of a behavior, a chaining procedure is utilized. There are two types of chaining procedures, forward and backward chaining. Backward chaining refers to a procedure in which the final behavior segment is taught first. This results in the client immediately completing the behavioral chain and receiving reinforcement for task completion. In forward chaining the first step of the task analysis is taught and then each subsequent step is added until the learner masters the entire sequence.

Each client will learn a new behavior at different rates, will need different types of prompts, will require prompts for varying lengths of time, and will respond to different reinforcers. In general, the degree of structure of the learning task, the number of prompts, and the amount of practice required for acquiring new behaviors will increase as the functioning level of the client decreases.

Exercises
9-2.   Define shaping and give an example of this technique in teaching a client a skill.
9-3.   Define the four types of prompts.
9-4.   Why is it necessary to fade prompts?
9-5.   Define imitation and suggest how it may be utilized to teach social skills.
9-6.   Define forward and backward chaining.

Answers to Exercises

9-2. Shaping refers to a procedure in which better and better approximations of the desired behavior are reinforced.

9-3. 1. Physical prompts, in which the staff member physically assists the client in performing a task.
2. Gestural prompts, in which the staff member gestures to the client how to perform a task.
3. Instructive prompts, in which the staff member provides verbal instruction to the client as to how to perform a task.
4. Imitative prompts, in which the staff member demonstrates the task.

9-4. Prompts are used to facilitate the acquisition of new behaviors. Prompts reduce the number of errors the client may make so that the behavior can occur correctly and be reinforced. The goal is to have the client perform the behavior independently and this requires that prompts be faded. Fading refers to the gradual removal of prompts.

9-5. Imitation, or modeling, refers to procedures in which clients learn new behaviors by observing others demonstrate the behaviors. This is particularly true if the clients have seen someone else being reinforced for performing a particular behavior.

Imitation is often useful in teaching appropriate social behaviors. Clients can observe staff and other clients engage in appropriate social behaviors. The staff and clients demonstrate the exact behaviors to be reinforced and the client imitates those behaviors.

9-6. Chaining refers to procedures in which discrete behaviors are combined into complex behaviors. A task analysis describes a chain of behaviors that when combined result in a complex behavior (i.e., hand washing as comprised of pushing up sleeves, turning on and adjusting water, wetting hands, and so forth).

Forward chaining refers to a procedure in which the discrete behaviors are taught from the beginning step to the final achievement of the complex behavior. The client is taught step 1 and then step 2 and so forth.

Backward chaining refers to a procedure in which the discrete behavior immediately preceding the final achievement is taught first. The next behavior taught is the behavior immediately preceding the behavior the client has mastered. A backward chaining program would begin with the final step of the task analysis.

SUGGESTED ACTIVITIES

1. Construct a task analysis for a simple motor skill such as assembling a ballpoint pen. After it is completed, ask a colleague to perform the steps as you read them from the task analysis. Keep notes on the performance and modify the task analysis as required.

2. Utilizing the modified task analysis, teach the skill to two clients. Use a forward chaining procedure with one client and a backward chaining procedure with the other client. Note the differences between the two procedures.

3. Clients may have difficulty in maintaining eye contact when they are speaking or being spoken to. Identify a client with a deficit in eye contact and use a shaping procedure to establish eye contact.

ADDITIONAL RESOURCES

Baker, B. L. *Behavior problems.* Champaign, Ill.: Research Press, 1976.

Cull, J. G., & Hardy, R. E. *Behavior modification in rehabilitation settings.* Springfield, Ill.: Charles C Thomas, 1974.

Gardner, W. I. *Behavior modification in mental retardation.* Chicago, Ill.: Aldine, 1971.

O'Leary, K. D., & O'Leary, S. G. *Classroom management, the successful use of behavior modification.* New York: Pergamon, 1972.

Rettig, E. G., & Paulson, T. L. *ABC's for teachers.* Van Nuys, Calif.: Associates for Behavior Change, 1975.

Sanders, R. M. *Behavior modification in a rehabilitation facility.* Carbondale, Ill.: Southern Illinois University Press, 1975.

Sulzer, B., & Mayer, G. R. *Behavior modification procedures with school personnel.* Holt, Rinehart, & Winston, 1972.

Sulzer-Azaroff, B., & Mayer, G. R. *Applying behavior procedures with children and youth.* New York: Holt, Rinehart, & Winston, 1977.

REFERENCES

Gagne, R. M. *The conditions of learning* (2nd ed.). New York: Holt, Rinehart, & Winston, 1970.

Gardner, W. I. *Learning and behavior characteristics of exceptional children and youth.* Boston: Allyn & Bacon, 1977.

Kazdin, A. *Behavior modification in applied settings.* Homewood, Ill.: Dorsey, 1975.

Moyer, J. R., & Dardig, J. C. Practical task analysis for special educators. *Teaching Exceptional Children,* 1978, *11,* 16-18.

Sloane, H. N., Buckholdt, D. R., Jenson, W. R., & Crandall, J. A. *Structured teaching.* Champaign, Ill.: Research Press, 1979.

Striefel, S. *Teaching a child to imitate.* Lawrence, Kans.: H & H Enterprises, 1977.

Chapter 10

Decreasing Behaviors

OBJECTIVES

To be able to:
1. Explain why programs designed to decrease excessive behaviors must always be paired with programs designed to promote adaptive behaviors.
2. Define reinforcement of alternative behaviors.
3. Define differential reinforcement of other behavior.
4. Define extinction.
5. Define timeout.
6. Define response cost.
7. Define overcorrection.
8. Describe advantages and disadvantages of each of the above procedures.

The use of procedures designed to decrease behaviors often raises legal and ethical issues. It is difficult to give many legal opinions on this subject because the implementation of procedures designed to decrease behaviors has been the focal point of many recent legal actions and ethical debates. According to Sloan, Buckholdt, Jenson, and Crandall (1979), legal decisions have reflected the following principles. Technically correct and ethical use of behavioral procedures that meet legal requirements is sound educational practice. Abuse of these procedures, as abuse of any approach, is often not only illegal and unethical but also counterproductive in habilitation. Concern for people, technical skill, and awareness of ethical standards and legal guidelines are prerequisites for success in using behavioral approaches.

The authors believe that the most appropriate way to deal with excessive behaviors is to design the environment so that the client does not have the opportunity to engage in excessive behaviors. Rather than focusing training efforts on decreasing behaviors, an alternative deficit in behavior should be identified and then subsequently reinforced. As the alternative behavior becomes more and more frequent, the excessive behavior will decrease and many times drop out altogether. For further information regarding the legal issues of behavior modification, interested readers are referred to Martin (1975).

EXCESSIVE BEHAVIORS

Excessive behaviors are inappropriate behaviors that oftentimes interfere with the performance of desired behaviors or with the acquisition of new behaviors, and that are viewed as undesirable (Gardner, 1977). Excessive behaviors are behaviors that need to be decreased. There are, however, several implications in implementing programs designed to decrease behaviors.

When reviewing the Individualized Program Plan and strengths/needs list of the client, we have often found that the majority of programs and goals listed are designed to decrease excessive behaviors. Although at times it is necessary to decrease behaviors, decreasing a behavior does not necessarily teach the client how to engage in appropriate behaviors. For example, if a client leaves his or her work station, setting up a program to decrease this behavior will not assure that the client will engage in a desired behavior such as working on task. The client may engage in a new undesired behavior. When decreasing an excessive behavior, it is essential to allow the opportunity for the client to engage in an appropriate behavior. In other words, you must plan for the replacement of excessive behaviors with appropriate behaviors.

Every excessive behavior is accompanied by a deficit in behavior. For example, a client who leaves his work station too much (excess) can also be viewed as a client who does not remain at his work station (deficit). The client who engages in a high rate of self-injurious behavior (excess) may have a deficit in working on task. It is difficult to engage in on-task behavior while engaging in self-injurious behavior.

This is the reason it is important to view excessive behaviors as having related deficits in behaviors. Behaviors in which there are deficits are increased through the use of positive reinforcement techniques and this results in teaching the client appropriate behaviors. Excessive behaviors are decreased by the use of procedures that do not necessarily teach appropriate behaviors.

The best way to reduce undesired behavior is to make desirable behavior so reinforcing that it successfully competes with undesired behavior (Sloane et al., 1979). It is therefore important to assess the learning environment to see if it optimizes the probability that desired behaviors will occur. Sloan et al. (1979) suggest that the analysis of the instructional setting should address the following questions:

1. Are the activities the most effective and motivating ones available? Do the activities relate to stated objectives or are they time fillers?
2. Does the organization of the training setting allow the instructor to work with individuals, small groups, and large groups as necessary?
3. Do the agency, program implementors, parents, and/or guardians feel that the activities are important?
4. Are preferred activities alternated with more difficult or nonpreferred activities?
5. Does the physical environment of the setting make it possible for the instructors to monitor clients and move easily about the room?
6. Is the pacing during presentation of materials and activities adequate to hold the client's attention?
7. Does the instructor use positive social reinforcement for desired behavior (is desired behavior rewarded in some way) and withhold attention for undesired behavior?

If the answer to any of these questions is "no," that area should be improved before implementing procedures designed to decrease behaviors. This is because instructional settings may contribute to the maintenance of excessive behaviors: peer attention may provoke and maintain excessive behavior, excessive behaviors may reflect deficits in certain aspects of self-control, the environment may be noisy or confusing, with many distractions such as clients walking around or bothering each other.

Exercise

10-1. Why is it important to view excessive behaviors as having related deficits in behavior?

Answer to Exercise

10-1. Deficits in behavior are changed through the use of positive reinforcement techniques, and this results in teaching the client appropriate behaviors. Excessive behaviors are decreased by the use of procedures that do not necessarily teach appropriate behaviors. Furthermore, if the client does not have the opportunity to engage in appropriate behaviors, the inappropriate behaviors may be replaced by other inappropriate behaviors.

INTERVENTION PROCEDURES

Many handicapped individuals have acquired a wide range of inappropriate behaviors that interfere with learning. Additionally, many of these inappropriate behaviors are strengthened by the consequences that they have produced. Intervention procedures that are designed to decrease or eliminate excessive behaviors include: 1) reinforcing alternative behaviors, 2) differential reinforcement of other behaviors, 3) extinction, 4) timeout, 5) response cost, and 6) overcorrection. The advantages and disadvantages of utilizing these procedures are shown in Table 10-1.

It is important to note that these procedures apply to both appropriate and inappropriate behaviors. For example, going to work is maintained by a pay check. How long would you go to work if you did not receive a pay check? This is an example of an extinction procedure that decreases behavior. Behavior is a function of consequences, and therefore may be increased, decreased, or maintained by its consequences.

Reinforcing Alternative Behaviors

Reinforcing alternative behaviors is a procedure in which reinforcement is provided for an explicit behavior or behaviors that are incompatible with the target behavior to be decreased (Gardner, 1977; Sulzer-Azaroff & Mayer, 1977). Reinforcing alternative behaviors provides positive reinforcement for the occurrence of an appropriate behavior that is incompatible with the behavior that is to be decreased.

A list of alternative behaviors that could be reinforced is shown below:

Inappropriate Behaviors	Alternative Behaviors
Off task	Working on task
Wandering around room	Staying at work station, sitting at table
Aggression, hitting, pushing	Interacting appropriately with others, appropriate assertiveness, requesting assistance, sharing materials, working on task
Noncompliance	Compliance with requests, cooperating with others, working on task

One of the authors worked with a profoundly retarded child who engaged in almost continuous hand clapping. A reinforcement procedure was implemented in which the child was reinforced for sitting in a chair with his hands in his lap. Having his hands in his lap was incompatible with hand clapping. As sitting with hands in lap increased, hand clapping decreased.

Basarich, Ferrara, and Rudrud (1980) utilized this procedure with severely emotionally disturbed adolescents in a self-contained classroom. The students engaged in a high rate of off-task behavior and a low rate of classwork completion. The program consisted of providing reinforcement for on-task behavior, which is incompatible with off-task behavior. There was a mean increase of 56.4% in on-task behavior and the mean number of assignments completed increased 91%.

Advantages of Reinforcing Alternative Behaviors   The major advantage of reinforcing alternative behaviors is that this is a positive and construc-

Table 10-1. Procedures for decreasing behaviors

Reinforcing Alternative Behaviors—Reinforcing an appropriate behavior that is incompatible with the excessive behavior.

Implementation	Advantages	Disadvantages
1. Alternative behavior must be incompatible. 2. Alternative behavior should be in the client's repertoire. 3. Alternative behavior should be practical and likely to be maintained through natural consequences of the environment. 4. Use positive reinforcement principles.	1. Positive approach. 2. Teaches appropriate behaviors. 3. Long-lasting.	1. May be a gradual reduction in the excessive behavior.

Differential Reinforcement of Other Behaviors (DRO)—Provide reinforcement on a regular schedule except following the occurrence of the excessive behavior.

Implementation	Advantages	Disadvantages
1. Schedule reinforcement carefully. 2. Reinforcement is provided for the nonoccurrence of a behavior. 3. Gradually and progressively increase the interval that the client must not engage in the excessive behavior.	1. Positive approach. 2. Long-lasting. 3. Rapid.	1. Reinforcement *must* be carefully scheduled. 2. "Other" behavior may be worse.

Extinction—Withholding reinforcement following the occurrence of the excessive behavior.

Implementation	Advantages	Disadvantages
1. Identify and control all reinforcers for the excessive behavior. 2. Maintain procedure long enough to show effect. 3. Be aware of temporary increase in behavior and spontaneous recovery.	1. Long-lasting. 2. When combined with positive reinforcement for alternative behaviors it is a positive approach. 3. Uncomplicated procedure.	1. Gradual. 2. May be temporary increase in response rate. 3. Spontaneous recovery may occur. 4. Sometimes difficult to identify and control reinforcers.

(continued)

Table 10-1. (continued)

Timeout—Removing the opportunity to earn reinforcement for X amount of time following the occurrence of the excessive behavior.

Implementation	Advantages	Disadvantages
1. Remove all reinforcers for a brief duration following occurrence of excessive behavior. 2. Make sure timeout is time out from positive reinforcement and is not being used as escape from training setting. 3. Administer timeout in matter-of-fact, nonemotional manner. 4. Be consistent and closely monitor timeout. 5. Arrange environment to prevent escape.	1. Long-lasting. 2. Rapid.	1. Physical movement of the subject may be necessary. 2. Time consuming. 3. May prompt escape and/or aggressive behavior. 4. Frequently misunderstood and therefore abused.

Response Cost—Withdrawing X amount of reinforcers contingent upon the occurrence of an excessive behavior.

Implementation	Advantages	Disadvantages
1. Allow for build-up of reinforcer reserve. 2. Communicate rules of the game. 3. Magnitude of response cost must "fit the crime."	1. Long-lasting. 2. Rapid. 3. Allows the client to stay in the training environment so that appropriate behaviors can be strengthened.	1. Effectiveness dependent upon client's reinforcement history. 2. May prompt escape and/or aggressive behavior.

Overcorrection—Correction procedure of two types:
1. Restitutional overcorrection, in which the responsibility for misbehavior is accepted by restoring the setting or situation to a vastly improved state.
2. Positive practice overcorrection, which requires the practice of appropriate modes of responding contingent upon episodes of inappropriate behavior.

Implementation	Advantages	Disadvantages
1. Overcorrection must be relevant to inappropriate behavior.	1. Forces correct practice. 2. Rapid.	1. Time consuming. 2. Physical restraint may be necessary.

(continued)

Table 10-1. (*continued*)

2. Apply immediately and consistently. 3. Arrange in environment to prevent escape. 4. Do not use excessive physical force when using positive practice.	3. Long-lasting. 4. Generalizes across settings and behaviors.	3. May not easily apply to all excessive behaviors.

tive approach. Since it is a positive reinforcing procedure, it increases appropriate behaviors. Remember, for every excessive behavior there is a related deficit. With this procedure, the client receives reinforcement for increasing appropriate behaviors. This is in sharp contrast to reductive procedures such as extinction, response cost, and timeout, which focus on eliminating behaviors. Decreasing behavior does not teach the client what to do; rather, it teaches what not to do.

Disadvantages of Reinforcing Alternative Behaviors Sulzer-Azaroff and Mayer (1977) indicate that one disadvantage with this procedure is that it takes time for the appropriate behavior to replace the inappropriate behavior. Until appropriate behavior is emitted at a fairly high rate, the client still has time available to engage in the inappropriate behavior.

Reinforcing Alternative Behaviors Effectively In selecting the alternative behavior, it is necessary to be very specific in choosing a behavior that is incompatible with the inappropriate behavior. For example, a client may leave his or her work station and, as a result, his or her production rate is lowered. Simply reinforcing staying at the work station may not increase the client's production. It is necessary to be very specific about which behaviors are to be reinforced.

It is also a good idea to select behaviors that are already in the client's response repertoire. If the behavior is not in the client's repertoire, it is necessary to utilize techniques designed to teach new behaviors. The intent of the procedure is to replace the inappropriate behavior with an appropriate behavior. This will be accomplished more rapidly if the appropriate behavior does not have to be taught.

Additionally, the alternative behavior should be practical. Practical behaviors are behaviors that are related to the client's habilitation plan, have social import, and are likely to be maintained through natural consequences in the environment. For example, if a client has temper tantrums, reinforcing sitting quietly in a chair is not the best alternative behavior. Rather, working is a behavior that is productive, practical, and most likely will be maintained by natural consequences.

Differential Reinforcement of Other Behaviors

Differential reinforcement of other behaviors (DRO) refers to a procedure in which reinforcement is delivered to the client as long as the client does not engage in the behavior to be eliminated. Reinforcement is contingent upon the nonoccurrence of a behavior. DRO is different from reinforcing alternative behaviors. In DRO reinforcement is delivered on a schedule for the *nonoccurrence* of a target behavior. Reinforcing alternative behaviors provides reinforcement for the *occurrence* of a behavior that is incompatible with the target behavior.

The DRO procedure is sometimes referred to as omission training. The authors utilized a DRO procedure in reducing the self-injurious behaviors of a profoundly retarded child. The child engaged in self-injurious behaviors such as hitting and biting himself and hitting his head against objects and in various other forms of self-mutilation at a rate of 45 responses per minute. The DRO procedure was implemented during mealtimes and consisted of providing a bite of food contingent on the nonoccurrence of self-injurious behavior. Initially, food was presented contingent on one-half second of no self-injurious behavior. As the training sessions progressed, food was contingent on 10 seconds of no self-injurious behavior. After three weeks, the rate of self-injurious behavior decreased to zero incidences per 20-minute mealtime.

Carroll, Sloop, Mutter, and Prince (1978) combined the use of DRO, satiation, and positive practice overcorrection to eliminate chronic clothes ripping in six severely or profoundly retarded individuals. Repp and Deitz (1974) reduced aggressive and self-injurious behaviors of four retarded children by combining various techniques with DRO procedures.

Advantages of DRO   DRO is a positive approach because the client receives positive reinforcement when not engaging in the target behavior. Additionally, since the client is not physically removed from the training session, the client has further opportunity to earn reinforcement for engaging in appropriate behaviors. DRO procedures produce rapid decrements in behavior and the results are very long lasting.

Disadvantages of DRO   DRO requires that reinforcement must be carefully scheduled. The reinforcement is scheduled so that the trainers know exactly when to deliver reinforcement. At first, the time interval for delivering reinforcement should be kept short, allowing the client to earn frequent reinforcement (Sulzer-Azaroff & Mayer, 1977). As the inappropriate behavior decreases in frequency, the intervals are gradually lengthened.

Another disadvantage that may occur is that the "other" behavior may be worse. The DRO procedure provides reinforcement to the client for engaging in an infinite variety of behaviors other than the specified target behavior. As a result, the client may be engaged in an inappropriate behavior that is not the target behavior when reinforcement is delivered. For example, if a DRO procedure is being utilized to decrease yelling, reinforcement is delivered on a schedule. The client may be engaged in another behavior such as body rocking or self-injurious behavior when reinforcement is to be delivered. This paradox is most likely to occur among clients who exhibit many problem behaviors. Sulzer-Azaroff and Mayer (1977) suggest that this problem can most effectively be dealt with by putting several of the more serious behaviors on DRO simultaneously or by utilizing another reductive procedure.

Extinction

Extinction refers to a procedure in which reinforcement is no longer presented after a behavior has occurred. As a result the behavior decreases. Ayllon and Michael (1959) decreased the amount of time a schizophrenic woman spent in the nurses' office. For two years, the woman had entered the nurses' office to talk with the nurses while the nurses attempted to work. The woman had been given instructions not to enter the work station, had been asked to leave, and had been led by the hand out of the office. Prior to the extinction procedure, the woman entered the work station an average of 16 times per day. The nurses' attention was a positive reinforcer and maintained her high frequency of visits. The nursing staff were taught to ignore the woman when she entered (extinction). By the seventh week, the number of times the woman entered the work station decreased to 2 per day.

Pinkston, Reese, LeBlanc, and Baer (1973) showed that teacher attention maintained a preschool child's aggression to his peers. The child's aggressive behavior was reduced when the teacher was instructed to ignore the child and attend to the peer or peers who were the target of the aggressive behavior.

As indicated by Sloane et al. (1979), in a classroom the most common reinforcer to be withheld during extinction is teacher attention. Teachers often assume that their commands to behave appropriately are punishing rather than reinforcing. Madsen, Becker, and Thomas (1968) investigated the effects of "sit down" commands on out-of-seat behavior. The more the teacher told out-of-seat students to sit down, the more often out-of-seat behavior occurred. Ignoring out-of-seat behavior resulted in its decrease. Thus, ignoring inappropriate behavior while showing approval for desired behavior was an effective method for controlling classroom behavior.

Extinction procedures become extremely effective when combined with positive reinforcement procedures. Liberman, Teigen, Patterson, and Baker (1973) worked with four schizophrenic patients with paranoid and grandiose delusions who had been hospitalized for an average of 17 years. During the baseline period, each patient was interviewed for four 10-minute sessions each day. The duration of rational speech before the onset of delusional speech during the 10-minute interviews was recorded. At the end of the day, the patients were allowed a 30-minute period to talk with a nurse-therapist while relaxing with coffee, snacks, and cigarettes. The procedure designed to decrease delusional speech consisted of two contingencies:

1. The 10-minute interview was terminated at the onset of delusional speech (extinction).
2. The amount of time for the evening chat and snacks was made directly proportional on a 1:1 ratio to the number of minutes of rational talk accumulated during the four daily interviews.

The amount of rational talk exhibited during the interviews increased from between 200% and 600% as the contingencies were introduced for each patient.

Advantages of Extinction   Extinction programs have several advantages over other procedures designed to decrease behaviors. The effects are long-lasting, it is an uncomplicated procedure, it is easy to implement, and it does not involve the use of aversive consequences.

Disadvantages of Extinction   There are several disadvantages involved in utilizing an extinction procedure. One disadvantage is that extinction procedures are not designed to strengthen adaptive behaviors. For example, when a client exhibits an inappropriate behavior, the instructor might ignore the behavior. By doing nothing more than ignoring, the instructor does not allow the client to engage in an appropriate behavior.

Another weakness is the fact that reinforcing events may be difficult to control. Oftentimes, the class clown engages in inappropriate behaviors such as making animal noises or throwing objects that are maintained by peer attention rather than the teacher's attention. If the teacher attempts to utilize an extinction procedure without the cooperation of the students in the classroom, the behaviors will most likely not decrease. One needs to have control over the reinforcers in order to withhold them.

When an extinction procedure is implemented, behavior may show a temporary increase in frequency and/or intensity. Allen, Turner, and Everett (1970) utilized an extinction procedure with a preschool child who exhibited tantrums. Prior to extinction, the child's tantrums had an average duration of 5 minutes. On the first day the extinction procedure was implemented, his first tantrum lasted 27 minutes followed by three additional tantrums which lasted 6 minutes, 3 minutes, and 1 minute, respectively. On the third day there was only one mild, 4-minute tantrum. By day four, no further tantrums occurred. Thus, an inappropriate behavior put on extinction may intensify before it gets better and it is necessary to maintain the extinction procedure long enough to obtain the effect.

An extinction procedure alone usually produces a gradual decrease in the behavior rather than a quick decline. If a quick decrease is desired, as with certain aggressive or self-injurious behaviors, it is necessary to combine an extinction procedure with other behavior change procedures or to use a different procedure altogether. As noted by Gardner (1977), the number of times a given behavior will occur after the positive reinforcers have been withdrawn is related to:

1. The number of times the behavior has been reinforced prior to the beginning of extinction.
2. The type and magnitude of previous reinforcing experiences.
3. The schedule of reinforcement previously provided.
4. The availability of alternative means of behaving that will produce the same or equally appealing reinforcers.
5. The relative value of the reinforcer at the time extinction is initiated.
6. The difficulty level of the behavior.
7. The level of assurance held by the person that reinforcement is no longer forthcoming following the behavior.

Another disadvantage of extinction procedures is a phenomenon known as spontaneous recovery. Spontaneous recovery refers to the reappearance of a behavior that has been extinguished. It is necessary for the instructor to continue to ignore the behavior because if the instructor does not, and attention was reinforcing, the behavior will be intermittently reinforced. Thus, the behavior will be more likely to occur again because intermittently reinforced behavior is more resistant to extinction.

Other disadvantages reported to occur with the use of extinction procedures include increase in emotional/aggressive behaviors and, unless positive behaviors are reinforced, the appearance of other undesirable behaviors.

Timeout from Positive Reinforcement

Timeout is a procedure in which the opportunity to earn reinforcers is removed for a brief period of time following the occurrence of an inappropriate behavior. During the usual implementation of this procedure, if a client engages in an inappropriate behavior, the client may be removed from the presence of the instructor and other peers and placed in a quiet room, office, corner, or other location that contains minimal objects, social stimulation, and opportunity for activities. The location is not important. What is important is that the timeout is time out *from positive reinforcement*.

In an elementary special education classroom, one of the authors implemented a timeout procedure in which if certain specified behaviors occurred a child was placed in timeout for 2 minutes. The child could return to the class if he or she was quiet for 2 minutes. The timeout area was a chair set behind a partition that was approximately 4 feet high. The teacher would

188 / Behavior Management

indicate who was to go to timeout, and the child would go to the timeout area and sit on the chair. The child could not see above the partition, and when timeout was over the teacher would tell the child to rejoin the class. As the program progressed, the number of times children were placed in timeout decreased from approximately 20 times per day to 1 or 2 times. Three weeks into the program, children went into timeout 40 times one morning. The teacher found that one of the children had "smuggled" a pen into the timeout area and one of the world's greatest murals was being completed. The children wanted to draw on the partition before it was filled up and, as a result, the timeout booth was positively reinforcing and children engaged in inappropriate behavior to continue drawing. During recess, the artists were required to wash the partition and the number of times children were required to go into timeout decreased to previous levels.

Sloane et al. (1979) have identified two types of timeout procedures: 1) timeout from positive reinforcement without isolation and 2) timeout from positive reinforcement with isolation. Timeout without isolation is utilized when the behavior is not harmful, dangerous, or disruptive to other people or is not self-destructive. This procedure was utilized when one of the authors worked with a client who engaged in inappropriate eating behaviors. At lunch and break times, the client would "stuff" all her food into her mouth rather than take appropriately sized bites and placing the food onto a plate. The client was instructed to take a piece of food, chew, and swallow the food before taking another piece. If the client attempted to take more than one piece or take a piece of food prior to swallowing, the instructor would take the plate and turn away from the client. The instructor would not turn back to the client until the client sat quietly for 30 seconds. After three weeks, the client was eating appropriately and cutting food into small bites.

The difference between timeout without isolation and extinction is that in extinction one specific behavior that has previously been reinforced is no longer reinforced. In timeout, no response is reinforced for a specified period of time following the occurrence of an inappropriate behavior (Sloane et al., 1979).

Timeout with isolation refers to a procedure in which the client is removed from the reinforcing environment. Most often this refers to a program in which the client is placed in a quiet room or removed from the presence of others. One way to think of this process is that using timeout with isolation is a way of boring the individual (Sloane et al., 1979). If a client exhibits an inappropriate behavior, the client is removed to an area where he or she will not disrupt others and where there is nothing to do. The client must remain in the timeout area until he or she is quiet for a brief period. Then the individual may return to regular activities.

In utilizing timeout procedures, the following guidelines are suggested:

1. Before utilizing timeout with isolation, try other procedures designed to decrease behaviors. Timeout is not a positive approach in that the client has no opportunity to be reinforced for appropriate behaviors while in timeout.

2. Closely monitor how often a client is placed in timeout (time, date, duration, reason, etc.) and how often the timeout area is utilized. Excessive use of timeout indicates that the training environment is not positively reinforcing. If the training environment was positively reinforcing, the clients would engage in high frequencies of appropriate behaviors.

3. Communicate to other staff and clients what behaviors will result in the implementation of the timeout contingencies. Consistency in program implementation is essential for decreasing behaviors. If a client is to be placed in timeout for hitting others, it is necessary to place the client in timeout no matter where the hitting occurs (e.g., in the lunchroom, in the shop, or in the classroom). By describing the behaviors that result in timeout to the clients, this specifies the relationship between these behaviors and the contingent consequences.

4. Administer timeout in a matter-of-fact, nonemotional manner. Scolding, reprimanding, and yelling at the client are to be avoided, as are requesting apologies, explaining why the client has to go into timeout, and praising the client for going into timeout.

5. Ensure that timeout is time out from positive reinforcement. Placing a client in the breakroom or supervisor's office may be quite reinforcing for the client. Needless to say, if a client is placed in timeout, other staff and clients should not interact with the client and the client should not be allowed snacks or cigarettes while in timeout.

6. Keep the timeout period short. Research has shown that timeout periods from 1 to 10 minutes have been effective (Gardner, 1977). Lengthy periods of timeout remove the client from the training environment, where he or she may learn appropriate behaviors. We have found that, when placed in timeout, the client should remain in timeout until he or she is quiet for 2 minutes. Thus, if the client tantrums for 5 minutes, he or she will remain in timeout for a total of 7 minutes.

Advantages of Timeout   A major advantage of timeout is that it is effective in reducing a wide variety of behaviors (e.g., temper tantrums, out-of-seat behaviors, off-task behaviors, hitting, spitting, verbal abuse, noncompliance). Timeout also produces fairly rapid decrements in behavior and it is a long-lasting procedure.

Disadvantages of Timeout   A disadvantage associated with the use of timeout is that timeout can be a time-consuming process. The benefits of decreasing the undesirable behaviors, however, usually outweigh this disadvantage. Other disadvantages are that physical movement of the client to timeout may be necessary and that escape behavior may occur.

Timeout can be abused for at least two reasons. People forget that timeout must be time out from reinforcement and that therefore the environment must be reinforcing for timeout to be effective. Also, it is not intended as a method for staff to escape via seclusion or isolation of the client.

Response Cost

Response cost refers to a procedure in which privileges, tokens, or other reinforcers are removed contingent upon the occurrence of specific inappropriate behaviors. In other words, inappropriate behaviors cost the client privileges, tokens, or other reinforcers. A familiar response cost procedure is that, if you are caught speeding, a sum of about $30 will be taken from you.

As with timeout, response cost has been used to decrease a wide variety of behaviors. Schmidt and Ulrich (1969) utilized a response cost procedure to decrease classroom noise and out-of-seat behavior of children. The children earned free time when they engaged in appropriate classroom behaviors but lost free time for inappropriate behavior. Other behaviors that have been reduced utilizing response cost procedures include: dysfluent speech, aggression, absenteeism, out-of-seat, smoking, overeating, stuttering, and psychotic talk (Kazdin, 1972; Sloane et al., 1979).

Advantages of Response Cost   Response cost procedures have been effective in reducing a wide variety of behavior in a variety of clinical settings. The procedure produces rapid decreases in behaviors that are long-lasting. It is usually easier and less disrupting to implement than timeout. Another advantage of response cost is that it allows the client to stay in the training environment, where appropriate behaviors can be reinforced.

Disadvantages of Response Cost   One disadvantage with response cost procedures is in determining the size of the fine. The client must have a reinforcer reserve. The fine should be large enough to decrease the behavior. Sloane et al. (1979) suggested that, if the fine removes half of the points or tokens, the fine is too large. On the other hand, if a client is fined many times during the day, the size of the fine is probably too small. It is necessary to provide the opportunity for the client to obtain the lost reinforcers. A special case occurs when the client has no reinforcers available. To implement a response cost procedure, the trainer should record the fine and collect the fine as soon as the client has reinforcers available. If the client is continually "in the hole," the response cost procedure will become ineffective in that reinforcement will never be obtained for appropriate behaviors. This can result in an "it doesn't matter" attitude. For example, suppose you are fined seven million dollars and you make minimum wage. How effective is the seven million dollar fine?

Overcorrection

Overcorrection is a procedure designed to decrease behaviors. It has two basic components: "1) to overcorrect the environmental effects of an inappropriate act, and 2) to require the disruptor to intensively practice overly correct forms of relevant behavior" (Foxx & Azrin, 1973, p. 2). The first component is called *restitutional overcorrection,* and requires the client to restore the environment to a better state than before the inappropriate behavior occurred. For example, if a client throws work materials, the client would be required to pick up and sort all of the materials and to dust and clean the area.

The second component is *positive practice overcorrection,* which involves repeated practice of a positive behavior. In the example of throwing work materials, the client would have to clean another client's work station. One of the authors worked with a client who would slam doors in a workshop and the workshop's van. During the positive practice overcorrection procedure, whenever the client would slam a door, regardless of location, the client was required to appropriately open and close the door 20 times. Door slamming was eliminated within two weeks.

Azrin and Powers (1975) utilized positive practice overcorrection to reduce disruptive classroom behaviors in a group of emotionally disturbed children. The children were informed of classroom rules of conduct. If a rule was broken, the child had to recite the infringed rule, practice and repeat the appropriate behavior for several trials, and engage in further positive practice during recess periods. Disruptive behavior was reduced 95%.

Agosta, Close, Hops, and Rusch (1980) utilized an overcorrection procedure to decrease hand biting by a preschool-age child. When the child bit his hand, the trainer gave a verbal reprimand following which the child had to brush his teeth with a toothbrush that had been soaked in an oral antiseptic (2-minute duration) and return to the training setting to take pegs from a pegboard and place them in a bowl (2-minute duration). Every time the child bit his hands, he was required to complete the entire procedure.

Advantages of Overcorrection   Overcorrection procedures have been applied to various behaviors and shown to produce rapid and long-lasting effects. Foxx and Azrin (1973) have found that overcorrection produces more rapid and long-lasting effects than other procedures.

Overcorrection is educational in that it teaches the client an appropriate behavior through practice.

Disadvantages of Overcorrection   One disadvantage of utilizing overcorrection is that it is a time-consuming procedure. Overcorrection must be instituted immediately following the occurrence of an inappropriate behavior. As a result, this usually requires an almost 1:1 staff/client ratio. Additionally, the client must engage in the overcorrection procedure for a set period of time.

Another difficulty is encountered when the client refuses to complete the overcorrection program. At this point, manual guidance is required and physical restraint may be needed.

Finally, the restitution activity must be relevant to the inappropriate behavior and, as a result, overcorrection may not easily apply to many behaviors. As stated by Sulzer-Azaroff and Mayer (1977), "What would be an appropriate restitution procedure for the behavior of peeking under a lady's skirt?" (p. 300).

Physical Punishment

Physical punishment and verbal threats were purposely not discussed as procedures to decrease behaviors. This is because at best these types of punishment only suppress behavior. In fact, as shown by Madsen, Becker, and Thomas (1968), the more the teacher told students to sit down, the higher the rate of out-of-seat behaviors. Other negative side effects that may occur include staff modeling inappropriate behaviors. Peer or other clients' reactions may pose a threat to the punished client (i.e., clients picking on the offender). Punishment may cause withdrawal, escape behavior, and/or aggression. Furthermore, these procedures are often abused, mostly when dealing with aggressive clients.

Observation has shown that too often a client's aggressive behavior is directly related to staff behavior. For example, one client was practicing pouring a beverage from a pitcher to a glass for other clients for the upcoming break. When the client was done, break time was announced, and the staff member informed the client that because of her morning performance she was not entitled to juice. When the staff member tried to remove the glass of juice, you can imagine the results. Other examples include when staff are in a hurry and begin herding clients to and from work areas. Pushing and prodding often begets pushing and prodding.

GUIDELINES IN USING BEHAVIORAL DECREMENT PROCEDURES

Regardless of which procedure is chosen to decrease inappropriate behaviors, the following guidelines are suggested.

1. *Evaluate environmental conditions.* Often inappropriate behaviors occur as a result of environmental conditions. One of the authors was asked to consult on a client who engaged in self-stimulatory behaviors. Observation revealed that the only time staff attended to the client was when the client engaged in the self-stimulatory behaviors. When the client worked or engaged in appropriate behaviors, staff did not reinforce the client.

2. *Be specific.* It is necessary to operationalize the behavior that is to be reduced. This is done so that all staff know that when client X does Y

then consequence Z must follow. This also means that consequence Z *only* occurs when client X does Y. When Sally complies with a request then she is reinforced. When Sally does not comply with a request, she is to be placed in timeout for 2 minutes. This means that all staff must know the contingencies and that if Sally tantrums or engages in another inappropriate behavior, she should not be placed in timeout unless the program is designed to deal with these behaviors.

3. *Be immediate.* The most effective learning occurs when positive or negative consequences immediately follow a behavior. It is important to establish the functional relationship that if X occurs then Y follows. A classic case in point is smoking. The threat of lung cancer has not decreased smoking. However, if a program was implemented in which every time you smoke a cigarette five dollars was subtracted from your paycheck, smoking would likely decrease.

4. *Be consistent.* If a client engages in an inappropriate behavior that is consequated inconsistently, it will take longer for the behavior to decrease. Additionally, a phenomenon known as behavioral contrast may occur. When an inappropriate behavior comes under stimulus control, it may be reduced under certain conditions but increased when the consequences do not follow. One study by the psychology department at Utah State Training School showed that when an aversive consequence was administered (contingent upon self-injurious behavior) by one staff member, self-injurious behavior decreased only in the presence of the particular staff member. When the staff member was not present, self-injurious behavior increased.

5. *Communicate the rules of the game.* When implementing programs to decrease behaviors, the specific behaviors that are to be decreased should be clearly communicated to the client. Posting the "rules" is helpful, particularly when using group consequences and/or response cost programs. Clear communicating of the rules helps to establish the functional relationship between behavior and its consequences.

SUMMARY

Clients often engage in inappropriate excessive behaviors that need to be reduced in order for the client to engage in appropriate behaviors. Procedures designed to decrease excessive behaviors include extinction, timeout, response cost, DRO, overcorrection, and reinforcing alternative behaviors. The authors maintain that most excessive behaviors can be decreased by reinforcing alternative behaviors. This is because excessive behaviors can be conceptualized as reflecting deficits in other behaviors. These other behaviors are increased through the use of positive reinforcement.

Exercises

10-2. Bill is a 35-year-old client who is working in the work adjustment program. Bill spends a considerable amount of time mumbling under his breath. Although this does not cause him much difficulty in his present setting, this behavior does distract other clients and labels Bill as different in more "normalized" settings (e.g., in the community, in competitive placement).

What alternative behaviors would you reinforce in Bill?

Why might this procedure be preferable to others?

10-3. Sally is a 23-year-old client who is working in the work adjustment program. When a supervisor gives instructions or criticism, Sally becomes sullen, closes her eyes, turns away from the instructor, and slows down in her work.

What are the excessive behaviors?

How would you deal with this problem?

10-4. John has recently moved into the group home. Previously he had lived with his elderly parents and had the run of the house—eating whenever he wanted, watching television all day, and never doing any chores. During the third night at the group home, John was asked to help wash the dinner dishes. He refused and sat in his chair watching television. When staff went to escort John to the kitchen, he jumped up, yelled at other clients, and began running through the home pushing and shoving staff and clients.

How would you deal with John's excessive behaviors?

Answers to Exercises

10-2. An alternative behavior to mumbling is being quiet. Reinforcing alternative behaviors is preferable for several reasons.

1. Extinction is a gradual procedure and the other clients are bothered by the mumbling.
2. DRO may be another method for decreasing mumbling; however, the "other" behaviors may be worse (i.e., wandering from work station, but being quiet).
3. Placing Bill in timeout may not reduce his mumbling in that he may mumble in timeout.
4. With overcorrection it may be difficult to specify an appropriate restitution procedure.
5. A response cost procedure would not be appropriate because a fine for an innocuous behavior is not warranted.

10-3. The excessive behaviors are turning away from the instructor and closing her eyes. Remember, excessive behaviors can be viewed as having related deficits in behavior. Behaviors Sally does not exhibit are looking at the instructor when being addressed, acknowledging criticism and/or instructions, remedying the situation, and maintaining adequate production rates. Most likely, in Sally's case, it would be necessary to teach these new behaviors rather than set up programs designed to decrease turning away.

10-4. John's behaviors need to be dealt with quickly. Since this is a fairly specific behavior, timeout or response cost would be the most appropriate type of program. It is necessary to provide reinforcement for engaging in appropriate behaviors so that John can learn alternative behaviors to these inappropriate behaviors.

SUGGESTED ACTIVITIES

1. Review a client's IPP. List the excessive behaviors that are addressed. Develop a list of deficits in behaviors to replace the excessive behaviors. Design a program to address these deficits.
2. List the advantages and disadvantages of procedures designed to decrease behaviors. Are there additional advantages and disadvantages that relate specifically to your setting and that will limit the utility of certain procedures (i.e., staff/client ratio, possible timeout areas)?
3. Select an excessive behavior that is to be decreased. Utilize the behavior problem analysis worksheet (see page 219) and implement a program to decrease this behavior.

ADDITIONAL RESOURCES

Adz, W. C., & Azrin, N. H. A comparison of several procedures for eliminating behavior. *Journal of the Experimental Analysis of Behavior*, 1963, *6*, 399-406.

Ayllon, T. Intensive treatment of psychotic behavior by stimulus satiation and food reinforcement. *Control of Human Behavior*, 1966, *1*, 170-176.

Azrin, N. H., & Weskowski, M. D. Theft reversal: An overcorrection procedure for eliminating stealing by retarded persons. *Journal of Applied Behavior Analysis*, 1974, *7*, 577-581.

Barton, E. S., Guess, D., Garcia, E., & Baer, D. M. Improvement of retardates mealtime behaviors by time out procedures using multiple baseline techniques. *Journal of Applied Behavior Analysis*, 1970, *3*, 77-84.

Becker, W. C., Madsen, C. H., & Thomas, D. R. The contingent use of teacher attention and praise in reducing classroom behavior problems. *Journal of Special Education*, 1967, *1*, 287-307.

Bostow, D. E., & Bailey, J. B. Modification of severe disruptive and aggressive behavior using brief timeout and reinforcement procedure. *Journal of Applied Behavior Analysis*, 1969, *2*, 21-38.

Burchard, J. D. Systematic socialization: A programmed environment for the habilitation of anti-social retardates. *Psychological Record*, 1967, *17*, 461-476.

Chiang, S. J., Iwata, B. A., & Dorsey, M. F. Elimination of disruptive bus riding behavior via token reinforcement on a distance based schedule. *Education and Treatment of Children*, 1979, *2*, 101-111.

Drabman, R. S., & Lahey, B. B. Feedback in classroom behavior modification: Effects on the target and her classmates. *Journal of Applied Behavior Analysis*, 1975, *7*, 591-597.

Emery, R. E., & Marholin, D., II. An applied behavior analysis of delinquency: The irrelevancy of relevant behavior. *American Psychologist*, 1977, *32*, 860-873.

Forehand, R., & Baumeister, A. A. Deceleration of aberrant behavior among retarded individuals. *Progress in Behavior Modification*, 1976, *2*, 223-278.

Foxx, R. M., & Azrin, N. H. Restitution: A method of eliminating aggressive-disruptive behavior of retarded and brain damaged patients. *Behavior Research and Therapy*, 1972, *10*, 15-27.

Guidry, L. S. Use of covert punishing contingency in compulsive stealing. *Journal of Behavior Therapy and Experimental Psychiatry*, 1975, *6*(2), 169-170.

Hamilton, J., Stephens, L., & Allen, P. Controlling aggressive and destructive behavior in severely retarded institutionalized residents. *American Journal on Mental Deficiency*, 1967, *71*, 852-856.

Haughton, E., & Ayllon, T. Production and elimination of symptomatic behavior. In

L. P. Ullman and L. Krasner (Eds.), *Case Studies in Behavior Modification.* New York: Holt, Rinehart, & Winston, 1965.

Holz, W. C., Azrin, N. H., & Ayllon, T. Elimination of behavior of mental patients by response-produced extinction. *Journal of Experimental Analysis of Behavior,* 1963, *4,* 407–412.

Kazdin, A. E. The effects of vicarious reinforcement on attentive behavior in the classroom. *Journal of Applied Behavior Analysis,* 1973, *6,* 71–78.

Kent, R. N., & O'Leary, K. D. A controlled evaluation of behavior modification with conduct problem children. *Journal of Consulting and Clinical Psychology,* 1976, *44,* 586–596.

Lewis, B. L., & Strain, P. S. Effects of feedback timing and motivational content on teachers' delivery of contingent social praise. *Psychology in the Schools,* 1978, *15,* 423–429.

Mithaug, D. E. A comparison of procedures to increase responding in three severely retarded, non-compliant young adults. *AAESPH Review,* 1979, *6,* 66–80.

Okavita, H. W., & Bucher, B. Attending behavior of children near a child who is reinforced for attending. *Psychology in the Schools,* 1976, *13,* 205–211.

O'Leary, K. D., & O'Leary, S. G. Ethical issues of behavior modification research in schools. *Psychology in the Schools,* 1977, *14,* 299–307.

Page, D. P., & Edwards, R. P. Behavior change strategies for reducing disruptive classroom behavior. *Psychology in the Schools,* 1978, *15,* 413–418.

Rose, T. L. Reducing self-injurious behavior by differentially reinforcing other behaviors. *AAESPH Review,* 1979, *4,* 179–186.

Schaefer, H. H., & Martin, P. L. *Behavioral therapy.* New York: McGraw-Hill, 1975.

Schutz, R. P., Rusch, F. R., & Lamson, D. S. Eliminating unacceptable behavior: Evaluation of an employer's procedure to eliminate unacceptable behavior on the job. *Community Services Forum,* 1979, *1,* 4–5.

Seinell, M. A., & Connis, R. T. Reducing inappropriate verbalizations of a retarded adult. *American Journal on Mental Deficiency,* 1979, *84,* 87–92.

Solomon, R. W., & Wahler, R. G. Peer reinforcement control of classroom problem behavior. *Journal of Applied Behavior Analysis,* 1973, *6,* 49–56.

Stumphauzer, J. S. Elimination of stealing by self reinforcement of alternative behavior and family contracting. *Journal of Behavior Therapy and Experimental Psychiatry,* 1976, *7,* 265–268.

Thomas, D. R., Becker, W. C., & Armstrong, M. Production and elimination of disruptive classroom behavior by systematically varying teacher's behavior. *Journal of Applied Behavior Analysis,* 1968, *1,* 35–45.

Ullmann, L. P., & Krasner, L. What is behavior modification. In L. P. Ullmann and L. Krasner (Eds.), *Case studies in behavior modification.* New York: Holt, Rinehart, & Winston, 1965.

Van Houten, R., & Van Houten, J. The performance feedback system in the special education classroom: An analysis of public posting and peer comments. *Behavior Therapy,* 1977, *8,* 366–370.

Wetzel, R. Use of behavioral techniques in a case of compulsive stealing. *Journal of Consulting and Clinical Psychology,* 1966, *30,* 367–374.

REFERENCES

Agosta, J. M., Close, D. W., Hops, H., & Rusch, F. R. Treatment of self-injurious behavior through overcorrection procedures. *Journal of the Association for the Severely Handicapped,* 1980, *5,* 5–12.

Allen, K. E., Turner, K. D., & Everett, P. M. A behavior modification classroom for Head Start children with problem behaviors. *Exceptional Children*, 1970, *37*, 119-129.

Ayllon, T., & Michael, J. The psychiatric nurse as a behavioral engineer. *Journal of the Experimental Analysis of Behavior*, 1959, *2*, 324-334.

Azrin, N. H., & Powers, M. A. Eliminating classroom disturbances of emotionally disturbed children by positive practice. *Behavior Therapy*, 1975, *6*, 525-534.

Basarich, T., Ferrara, J., & Rudrud, E. Validation of the PSMP with severely emotionally disturbed adolescents. Unpublished manuscript, University of South Dakota, 1980.

Carroll, S. W., Sloop, E. W., Mutter, S., & Prince, P. L. The elimination of chronic clothes ripping in retarded people through a combination of procedures. *Mental Retardation*, 1978, *16*, 246-249.

Foxx, R. M., & Azrin, N. H. The elimination of autistic self stimulatory behavior by over correction. *Journal of Applied Behavior Analysis*, 1973, *6*, 1-10.

Gardner, W. I. *Learning and behavior characteristics of exceptional children and youth*. Boston: Allyn & Bacon, 1977.

Kazdin, A. E. Response cost: The removal of conditioned reinforcers for therapeutic change. *Behavior Therapy*, 1972, *3*, 73-82.

Liberman, R. P., Teigen, J., Patterson, R., & Baker, V. Reducing delusional speech in chronic paranoid schizophrenics. *Journal of Applied Behavior Analysis*, 1973, *6*, 57-64.

Madsen, C. H., Becker, W. C., & Thomas, D. R. Rules, praise and ignoring elements of elementary classroom control. *Journal of Applied Behavior Analysis*, 1968, *1*, 139-150.

Martin, R. *Legal challenges to behavior modification*. Champaign, Ill.: Research Press, 1975.

Pinkston, E. M., Reese, N. M., LeBlanc, J. M., & Baer, D. M. Independent control of a preschool child's aggression and peer interaction by contingent teacher attention. *Journal of Applied Behavior Analysis*, 1973, *6*, 115-124.

Repp, A. C., & Deitz, S. M. Reducing aggressive and self-injurious behavior of institutionalized retarded children through reinforcement of other behaviors. *Journal of Applied Behavior Analysis*, 1974, *7*, 313-325.

Schmidt, G. W., & Ulrich, K. E. The effects of group contingent events upon classroom noise. *Journal of Applied Behavior Analysis*, 1969, *2*, 171-179.

Sloane, H. N., Buckholdt, D. R., Jenson, W. R., and Crandall, J. A. *Structured teaching*. Champaign, Ill.: Research Press, 1979.

Sulzer-Azaroff, B., & Mayer, G. R. *Applying behavior analysis procedures with children and youth*. New York: Holt, Rinehart, & Winston, 1977.

Chapter 11

Maintenance and Generalization of Behavior Change

OBJECTIVES

To be able to:

1. Explain why it is important to program for maintenance and generalization of behavior change.

2. Give four guidelines for promoting maintenance and generalization of behavior change.

3. Give two uses of antecedent conditions to promote maintenance and generalization of behavior change.

4. Give three uses of consequences that promote maintenance and generalization of behavior change.

5. Describe the ways in which self-management can be used to promote maintenance and generalization of behavior change.

6. Design a behavioral program that uses the guidelines and techniques described in this chapter to promote maintenance and generalization of behavior change.

How many times have you or one of your co-workers complained that you have taught an individual a new skill but, when it comes time for the person to use it, he or she doesn't seem to be able to remember what to do? How many times have you heard someone say "Judy was doing so well on that program, but now she's not working as hard anymore and I don't understand why"? These problems result from failure to achieve maintenance and generalization of behavior change. Such problems are almost universal. In a recent review of behavior modification programs in community-based settings, O'Donnell (1977) found that in nearly all cases improvements made while programs were in effect were not maintained after the participants left programs or after the behavior change programs were terminated.

Maintenance and generalization of positive behavior changes are absolutely necessary in order for these changes to be meaningful. An individual who has been taught how to work at a competitive rate but who is not capable of maintaining that rate over time is not going to be able to hold down a job. The person who knows how to cook dinner only on the stove in the group training home where he or she resides is not going to be able to feed himself or herself in an apartment. Furthermore, one of the strongest findings of the applied research done in this area is that the "train and hope" approach to maintenance and generalization is not very effective (Stokes & Baer, 1977). The train and hope strategy refers to establishing a behavior modification program that results in the learning of the desired behaviors and then ending the program and hoping that the behaviors will continue to occur over time and will occur in the desired locations. Hope is not sufficient. Instead, it is necessary to systematically plan for maintenance and generalization of behavior change, but only after the behavior has reached acceptable levels.

Before proceeding any further, let's stop to define our terms. By maintenance, or more specifically response maintenance, we refer to the continued occurrence of a behavior over time. In other words, we want the behavior to maintain over a long period of time. The type of generalization we will be discussing in this chapter is referred to as stimulus generalization. Stimulus generalization refers to the occurrence of a behavior under stimulus conditions that are different in some way from the conditions in which the behavior was trained. These conditions might differ with respect to place, physical structure, people present, noise level, and so forth. For instance, an individual who must learn to dress herself must be able to get dressed using a variety of clothing.

It is usually necessary to teach generalization because it is well known that behavior is situation specific (Marholin, Siegel, & Phillips, 1976). That is, most people learn to display behaviors they have acquired only in the situations in which the behaviors were learned. Think about all the ways that you behave in some places that you don't behave in other places. Throwing peanut shells on the ground at a baseball game is appropriate, but most people wouldn't even think about throwing their peanut shells on the floor of a fancy restaurant. What we know about the principles of learning tells us that discrimination is more likely to occur than generalization (Holman, 1977). We are more likely to learn that it is only acceptable to behave in a certain way in a limited number of locations than we are to learn that it is alright to behave that way in lots of different locations. This is particularly true of individuals who have been labeled as mentally retarded. One of the traditional descriptions of such individuals is that these people are unable to use previously learned skills in new situations (Langone & Westling, 1979).

Teaching generalization is difficult because inappropriate behaviors are just as likely to generalize as appropriate behaviors unless programs are very carefully designed to avoid this (Sulzer & Mayer, 1972). As Langone and Westling (1979) have observed, we don't want an individual who learns to hammer with a hammer to also hammer with a screwdriver. We do, however, want that person to be able to hammer with different types of hammers in different types of situations.

GUIDELINES FOR PROMOTING MAINTENANCE AND GENERALIZATION

Train Significant Others

One common recommendation that is made for promoting maintenance and generalization of behavior change is that individuals whom the client sees on a regular basis be taught programming techniques that will support the desired behaviors (Kazdin, 1975; Gardner, 1977). Significant others are the people we see most often, the people we live and work with. Training significant others usually means training parents, roommates, work supervisors, or teachers. This assures that consequences for behavior are carried out in the natural environment.

We recommend teaching significant people in the client's everyday environment to support behavior change only as an intermediate measure for two reasons. One is that the principles of learning apply to everyone. We then have to ask, suppose we teach the people in a person's environment to reinforce the occurrence of the behavior—then who reinforces the reinforcers (O'Donnell, 1977)? That is, if we train significant others to carry out behavior change programs we have to worry about who is reinforcing the significant others for reinforcing clients. The other reason that we only recommend training significant others as an intermediate measure is that ultimately people need to learn to control their own behavior if they are going to become independent members of the community.

Teach Functional Behaviors

One of the questions we constantly need to ask ourselves as we design programs and choose goals is: what is the purpose or function of the behavior that I am teaching? It is not functional just to teach people how to ride a city bus. It is functional to teach them how to ride a bus only if we teach them how to use that knowledge to get to work, to get to a movie, to go grocery shopping, to get to a friend's house, and so forth. It is not functional to teach people how to subtract three-digit numbers unless those three-digit numbers mean something. It is functional to teach people how to do enough three-digit addition and subtraction so that they can prepare a budget based on their income.

Probably the functional behavior that is the most difficult to teach is how to solve a problem. This is not really a functional behavior but rather a series of them. For instance, one of the authors worked with a young man who had been taught how to cross the street safely at a stop light. One day the people who worked with him went out looking for him when he was three hours late coming home from work. They found him standing at an intersection waiting for the stop light to turn green. The light was broken and it had been temporarily changed to a flashing red. It had not turned green and was not going to for quite some time. This young man had not learned what to do when something unexpected or unusual happened that upset his daily routine. It is therefore extremely important that we teach people how to identify problems and how to either solve them or get help solving them.

Teach Behaviors Clients Want to Learn

Usually when people want to learn a particular skill it's because they want to use that skill. Therefore, teaching them skills that they want to learn increases the likelihood that they are going to use the skills that they learned. This seems so obvious that it's almost silly to say it. Most of us, as much as we are able, chose the things that we wanted to learn in school and chose the kinds of jobs that we have because they are the kinds of jobs that we like to do. Now obviously this isn't always possible for all people at all times. It is not possible to teach someone who reads at the third grade level to be an airplane pilot. However, too often clients are discouraged from trying to acquire skills they are interested in, not because they're not capable of acquiring those skills, but because the agency doesn't have the necessary resources to teach them. When it is lack of resources that prevents us from teaching people the skills they want to learn, we need to try to find the appropriate resources (described in Chapter 17) somewhere else rather than simply discouraging clients.

Teach Clients Behavior Management

In order to become an independent member of the community, an individual must be able to control his or her own behavior to some extent and to have some effect on the behavior of other people. Thus, probably the most important guideline for promoting maintenance and generalization of behavior change is that individuals should be taught to manage their own behavior. Specific components and procedures for teaching self-management are discussed in another section of this chapter. Additionally, we all need to know to some extent how to be able to affect other people's behavior. This may be something as simple as being able to call and order pizza delivered to the door or it may be as complex and important as getting your work supervisor to pay attention to you and provide you feedback on how you are doing on the job. We therefore need to take a look at whether the individuals we serve are aware of how their behavior affects other people and how they can use their behavior to affect the ways in which others relate to them.

Exercises

11-1. 1. Define maintenance.
       2. Explain why programming for maintenance is an important part of behavior programming.
11-2. 1. Define generalization.
       2. Explain why programming for generalization is an important part of behavior programming.
11-3. Describe the four guidelines for designing maintenance and generalization programs. Take each guideline and explain why a program consistent with this guideline will promote maintenance and/or generalization.

Answers to Exercises

11-1. 1. Maintenance refers to the continued occurrence of a behavior over time.
       2. People who do not maintain their behavior over time are not likely to succeed as independent members of a community.
11-2. 1. Generalization refers to the occurrence of a behavior under conditions that differ in some way from the conditions under which the behavior was learned.
       2. Behaviors tend to occur only in the situations where they are learned.
11-3. Train significant others.
       Teach functional behaviors.
       Teach behaviors clients want to learn.
       Teach clients behavior management.

TECHNIQUES FOR PROMOTING MAINTENANCE AND GENERALIZATION

Techniques Involving Antecedents

We can think of generalization as having two different levels. The first level is the kind of generalization we want to get so that behaviors will occur under a variety of different conditions within a training program (Martin & Pear, 1978). For instance, we may want a behavior such as compliance to occur in the presence of a variety of different people. The second level of generalization is generalization from the training program to the natural environment (Martin & Pear, 1978). For instance, we will want work behaviors that we've trained to generalize from the training situation to a regular job. The two specific techniques that we are going to present for using antecedents to promote generalization are directly tied to these two levels. The first technique is to vary training conditions, the second is to equate stimulus conditions with the natural environment.

Varying Training Conditions   The people who write about varying training conditions sometimes refer to this as training sufficient examples (Stokes & Baer, 1977). It is often necessary to teach people to perform behaviors in many different examples of the conditions under which these behaviors have to occur. Most of the research in this area has looked at the need to train behaviors in the presence of several different trainers if generalization is to occur (Stokes & Baer, 1977). Some of the other conditions that you may want to vary during training are noise level, time of day, materials, number of other people present, sex of other people present, age of other people present, and specific wording of instructions given (Langone & Westling, 1979). In general, what you need to do is analyze all of the conditions under which the behavior should occur and then provide as many different conditions as possible and as many different combinations as possible during your training. To put it another way, you need to analyze the various types of cues that exist for this behavior in order to make them part of your program (O'Donnell, 1977). As you do this keep in mind Martin and Pear's (1978) caution that behavior should be established successively in different situations from the easiest to the most difficult. This is a commonsense kind of caution. You may want someone to be able to work while other people are present, but that doesn't mean you have to start training in a group. You may want someone to perform a skill while there is a radio blaring in the background, but that doesn't necessarily mean that you have to start training with the radio going. Make sure you have the behavior under control before you start bringing in a lot of distractors, even if those distractors will ultimately be part of the conditions under which the behavior must occur.

Equate Stimulus Conditions with the Natural Environment One of the most common recommendations given for promoting generalization of behavior to natural environments is to make training conditions as much like the natural environment as possible (Kazdin, 1975; Stokes & Baer, 1977; Martin & Pear, 1978). This is because the more the training situation is like the natural situation, the more likely it is that the behavior that was learned in the training situation will generalize (Kazdin, 1975). Making the training environment as much like the natural environment as possible is not quite as easy as it sounds. There are two reasons for this. First, there is no such thing as *the* natural environment. Rather, there are many natural environments. Teaching someone to buy their groceries in one particular supermarket in a community is a good example of this problem because in most communities there are several supermarkets to choose from.

The other difficulty we are faced with when we attempt to make training conditions as much like the natural environment as possible is that we must decide which cues in the natural environment are important. For instance, when we teach someone to cross the street does it matter how many other people there are making the crossing at the same time? When we teach someone to run a washing machine in a laundromat does it matter what color the washing machine is? Probably not, but we don't always know which cues people will attend to and which ones they won't. However, it is possible to identify some of the important cues that we find in a community and then make those cues part of our training program.

A recent article by Nutter and Reed (1978) described a program to teach color coordination and clothing selection to profoundly and severely retarded women. The color coordination choices were based on choices found in the community. Specifically, observers made records of the most common color combinations found at an indoor shopping mall, at a restaurant, and on a downtown sidewalk for a total of over 12½ hours of observation. The women being trained were then taught to select common color combinations when they selected clothes to wear. Neef, Iwata, and Page (1978) constructed a simulated model of several city blocks in a classroom for use in teaching bus riding skills. The model included buildings, traffic signals, dolls, slides, and a simulated bus. Both of these programs taught skills that were acceptable and useful in the community surrounding the training programs.

Exercises

11-4. What are the two ways this section gave for using antecedent conditions to promote maintenance and generalization?
11-5. Suppose you are teaching someone how to wet-mop a floor. How would you use the guidelines and techniques given in this chapter so far to promote generalization of floor mopping skills?
11-6. Suppose you are teaching a class in how to do grocery shopping. How would you use the procedures given in this section for promoting generalization to increase the likelihood that your students will be able to shop in stores in your community?

Answers to Exercises

11-4. Varying training conditions.
Equating stimulus conditions with the natural environment.
11-5. Vary type of mop used, type of floor mopped, who does the training, size of room mopped, shape of room mopped, type of supplies (e.g., soap) used, location of supplies, building where mopping occurs.
11-6. Vary store used to teach in, type of items bought, number of items bought, time of day shopping occurs.

Use of Consequences

We can only expect a behavior to occur where we want it to if there are consequences that will maintain the occurrence of the behavior in the desired setting (Marholin et al., 1976). In other words, we cannot expect a behavior to be maintained in the natural environment unless it is reinforced in the natural environment. This section discusses three techniques for the programming of consequences that are likely to result in the maintenance of behavior.

Use of Naturally Occurring Consequences Numerous authors have recommended that naturally occurring consequences are needed in order to promote the maintenance of behavior (Kazdin, 1975; Stokes & Baer, 1977; Martin & Pear, 1978). Naturally occurring reinforcers are reinforcers for behaviors that occur in the environments where you want the behaviors to occur. Some typical naturally occurring reinforcers in work situations are feedback and/or praise about performance, special assignments, company parties, friendly interactions with other employees, jobs with more responsibility, extended breaks, and the use of company time for personal projects (Luthans & Kreitner, 1975). Naturally occurring reinforcers outside of work may include favorite foods, television, romantic attention, sleeping late, phone calls from friends, clothes, movies, compliments in public, verbal praise in general, or going out to eat (Hall, 1975).

When you program for the use of naturally occurring reinforcers to maintain behavior there are three cautions you need to keep in mind. First, a reinforcer is only a reinforcer for a specific individual if it maintains that individual's behavior. In other words, just because a particular consequence maintains most people's behavior, don't assume that it maintains everyone's behavior. Second, there is no single natural environment; rather, there are many natural environments. Make sure that the naturally occurring reinforcers you choose really do occur in the relevant environments. Finally, many developmentally disabled individuals are not reinforced by those things that we typically consider naturally occurring reinforcers. That is, there may well not be sufficient reinforcement available in the natural environment to maintain those individual's behaviors (Stokes & Baer, 1977). You may therefore find it necessary to pair consequences that you would like to become reinforcing for a particular individual with consequences that are already reinforcing for that person.

One natural consequence that is often paired with existing reinforcers is verbal praise. For instance, Dorow (1980) paired verbal approval with music and with music and food in order to condition both music and approval as reinforcers for a severely retarded nonverbal 15-year-old woman. This type of program can be extremely effective if the pairing occurs many times over many days in order to give lots of exposure to the pairing. It is also a good idea once the new reinforcer has become effective to occasionally present it paired with the original reinforcer so that it will maintain its reinforcing properties.

Thin Schedules of Reinforcement It is well known that behavior is more likely to persist under intermittent reinforcement conditions (Sulzer & Mayer, 1972). Most of us are not reinforced very consistently or very often for much of our behavior. However, most of us continue to behave in expected ways at home and at work very consistently even though we are on thin, or lean, intermittent schedules of reinforcement. For most of the people you work with, in order to end up with behavior that is maintained on a thin intermittent schedule of reinforcement you,will need to plan to gradually reduce the amount, frequency, and consistency of reinforcement over time. This is because most of your training programs will start out with fairly frequent, often continuous schedules of reinforcement. This is exactly as it should be. You should not attempt to teach a new behavior using a very thin schedule of reinforcement. That comes later after you have established the behavior.

The key word to remember when making the change from the continuous type of schedule that is usually used for training to the thin intermittent schedule that you want for maintenance is *gradual*. If you start to thin a schedule of reinforcement and the behavior you're interested in maintaining starts to drop off, that probably means you are removing reinforcement too quickly. You need to back up and thin the schedule more gradually. Ideally, your end goal should be to have the behavior maintained on a schedule that is as much as possible like the schedule that occurs in the natural environment. There will, of course, be some practical limitations to how much like natural schedules your schedules can be. Obviously, you need to choose a schedule of reinforcement that is convenient to administer. A schedule that is very much like the naturally occurring schedule will not be effective if it is too complicated for you and your colleagues to use practically as part of your daily routine.

Increase Delays in Reinforcement Reinforcers that are part of daily life frequently are not presented immediately after the occurrence of the behavior being reinforced. Hence, to set up a program that approximates natural conditions you will need at some point to gradually increase the delay between the occurrence of the desired behavior and the presentation of the reinforcer for it (Kazdin, 1975). Probably the most common real-life examples of delays in reinforcement are pay schedules. Most people who work for a living are paid either once a week, once every two weeks, or once a month. That means you are expected to display a large quantity of work behavior over a fairly long period of time before being paid for it. Although it is hoped that most of us have other reinforcers operating for our work behavior in addition to the pay check, at some point we all needed to learn that that particular reinforcer was going to be presented regularly on a very delayed basis. The clients you work with will need to learn that same thing if they are going to become independent members of the community.

Earlier we discussed the differences between programming for generalization within the training environment and programming for generalization from the training environment to the natural environment. We can make the same kind of distinction between programming for maintenance within the training situation and from training to the natural environment. Making the move from the training situation to the situation where a behavior is supposed to occur can be somewhat disruptive to what have been previously consistent and reliable patterns of behavior. In order to increase the likelihood that behavior will continue to occur at the desired level after a move to the natural environment, you need to see that the behavior is reinforced somewhat more frequently in the new environment than it has been in the training environment. There are two different ways to go about doing this. One is to add new reinforcers to the natural environment and then gradually fade them out to help support the behavior during the initial transition. The other approach is to gradually reduce the frequency and consistency of reinforcement in the training program until the individual is receiving less reinforcement than what the natural environment will provide. Then when the move is made to the natural environment the amount of reinforcement for the desired behavior will be greater than what it has been in the training setting (Martin & Pear, 1978).

Exercises

11-7. Give at least two examples of naturally occurring consequences that maintain normal work behavior.

11-8. Give at least two examples of behaviors you regularly display at home that are maintained on thin schedules of reinforcement.

11-9. Give at least two examples of your behavior that are typically reinforced after a considerable delay.

Answers to Exercises

11-7. Examples might include: compliments, coffee breaks, smiles, a bonus, extra time off, a promotion, a raise in pay.

11-8. Answers to this will be different for different people. Some possibilities are: cleaning your house, weatherstripping windows, planting flower or vegetable seeds.

11-9. For most people an example of delayed reinforcement is your pay check. Other possibilities are: letters from friends in response to your letters, insurance claims (a reinforcer for paying premiums).

Teach Self-Management

Everyone who is considered an independent member of the community manages his or her own behavior to some extent. Most of us manage to get up in the morning, see that we are properly fed and cleaned, see that our houses or apartments are relatively clean, and get to work when we are supposed to be there without other people cuing us and reinforcing us every step of the way. If the clients we serve are going to be able to do these things, at some point we need to start teaching them to manage their own behavior. In this section we briefly describe self-management of both antecedents and consequences.

Self-Management of Antecedents Managing antecedents involves altering stimuli that happen just before behavior is to occur. There are at least three ways in which we all manage the antecedent cues for our own behavior. We tell ourselves what to do, we arrange cues in our environment that remind us to do things, and we ask others to provide cues for us. The process of telling oneself how to systematically solve a problem is usually called self-instruction. Programs designed to teach self-instruction are often similar to the one described by Gardner (1977). First the teacher acted as a model in performing the task while the child watched and the child performed the same task while the teacher provided instruction. Then the child was asked to repeat the task while saying the instructions to himself or herself. Finally, the child completed the task while whispering the instructions and then completed the task while not saying the instructions audibly but presumably saying them to himself or herself. Consider what the self-instructions might sound like if you were teaching someone how to follow a recipe. "Let's see, first I have to read the recipe. The first thing the recipe says to do is to turn on the oven to 350°. Okay, I've done that. Now it says these are ingredients, I guess I better get out the ingredients . . ." and so forth.

We all provide ourselves with multiple cues in our environments that help remind us to do things. Most people set an alarm clock in order to have a cue for when it's time to wake up to go to work. Many of us use shopping lists to provide cues for what we need to buy at the grocery store. We all need to learn what cues we need in order to function effectively on a daily basis. Whereas some cues, such as alarm clocks, are used by nearly all members of society, others are only needed by a few of us. You will need to help the people you work with learn how to use whatever cues they require in order to function effectively.

The last way of using self-management to arrange antecedents is to have other people provide cues. When we ask friends to remind us to do something we are managing the cues in our environment. Whenever we ask a dentist to call and remind us when it's time for another checkup we are arranging the cues for ourselves. Once again, this type of self-management is a skill that can be taught to the people we serve.

Self-Management of Consequences Self-management of consequences is management of what happens after a behavior occurs. It can be thought of as having at least four parts: self-reporting of behavior, self-evaluation of behavior, self-determination of consequences, and self-administration of those consequences (Gardner, 1977). It is important to remember here, as we talk about teaching each of these four steps, that as you teach each step you will need to reinforce its occurrence initially. This is particularly true before you get to the stage of teaching self-delivery of consequences. The development of self-management skills is a gradual process like the learning of any new behavior and must initially be supported by outside consequences like any other behavior. An individual cannot be expected to manage his or her own behavior unless he or she knows what that behavior is. Hence, the first stage to developing self-management skills with respect to consequences is developing the skills to record your own behavior. Sometimes mere recording of your own behavior is sufficient to change it (Martin & Pear, 1978). For instance, many people who begin a program to manage their eating or smoking behavior cut down on their food or cigarette consumption when they discover how much they really eat or smoke in a day. The biggest problem with self-recording is that sometimes it is not very accurate. Hence, when you teach self-recording it is important to reinforce accurate self-reporting of behavior (Stokes & Baer, 1977).

The next stage in learning to self-manage consequence delivery is the development of skills in evaluating your own behavior. In our experience the people we serve have often not learned how to evaluate their own behavior. They frequently do not know how to tell when they have done a good job on a particular task. Sometimes they don't even know when they are finished doing the task. These are problems of learning to discriminate between when a task is done or not done, or when a job is done well or is not done well enough. In order to be able to teach this type of discrimination you will need to be able to identify the standard for deciding when a behavior is acceptable and when it is not.

The third stage in self-management of consequences is learning to decide what the appropriate consequence is for a particular behavior. In order to do this you have to know what consequences you have under your control and are therefore able to deliver. The one thing that most of us have at least some control over is how we use our time. How many times have you said to yourself "I'm not going to read that new murder mystery until I've finished studying for the exam tomorrow," or "I'm not going to relax in front of the television until I've finished painting the kitchen." These are examples of people making decisions about what consequences to deliver contingent on certain behaviors.

The final step in learning to self-manage consequences is learning to deliver your own reinforcement when you have earned it. This can range all the way from saying to yourself "Hey, I did a good job" to taking yourself out to dinner, calling a friend, going to a football game, or curling up with a good book.

All of these self-management procedures have been successfully taught to developmentally disabled individuals. Connis (1979), for example, taught four mentally retarded adults to cue themselves to proceed from one job task to the next by making an X on a picture of the next task to be performed and then beginning work. Three months after the program ended these individuals were still proceeding from task to task and using the self-cuing procedures. Shapiro and Klein (1980) taught four moderately retarded children, ages 6 to 9, to maintain their own on-task behavior by teaching them to first discriminate whether or not they were on task. Second, the instructor gradually faded out verbal prompts so that the children were evaluating whether they were on task themselves. Third, the children were taught to reinforce themselves with tokens for remaining on task for a set period of time. Finally, they were taught to reinforce themselves without a prompt. These children were still maintaining high levels of on-task behavior 8 weeks after programming ended.

The research on how to teach self-management procedures is still sketchy and a great deal more work is needed, but the results that are available are extremely encouraging.

Exercises

11-10. Describe at least six examples of ways in which you use antecedents to manage your own behavior. For each example you give tell whether it is an example of giving yourself instructions, arranging your environment, or asking others to help you cue yourself.

11-11. Take two examples of your own behavior that you self-manage with consequences. For each of these examples describe how you observe the behavior, how you evaluate whether or not it is satisfactory and how you deliver the consequences for it.

Answers to Exercises

11-10. Only you know the answers to this one. How do your answers compare to those of your co-workers?

11-11. Again, only you know the answers to this one. Compare your answers to those of your co-workers.

A FINAL COMMENT

The purpose of this chapter was to provide you with some general guidelines and specific techniques for writing programs that will promote appropriate maintenance and generalization of behavior change. However, we would like to add one note of caution. As a result of the increase in the types and numbers of services available, many developmentally disabled individuals are frequently moved from institutions to a variety of community-based facilities, or from facilities in one community to those in another community, or from their parents' home to a group home. Making a major change in our living or working situation is pretty unsettling for most of us. The move from an institution to a group home has been compared by Coffman and Harris (1980) to the aftermath of divorce or release from prison. People who have been through that kind of a major change in their lives generally need a chance to adjust. So, do use the guidelines and procedures we have described to plan for maintenance and generalization, but don't jump in and use them immediately after someone has just made a major move. Give them a chance to adjust first. After all, most of us don't immediately start doing everything we're capable of the minute we move into a new home or a new job.

SUGGESTED ACTIVITIES

1. Pick a client you work with regularly, and read through this client's current programs. Ask yourself whether these programs are designed to promote maintenance and generalization of behavior change. If not, propose changing them so that they do.

2. Pick the client you work with regularly who is closest to becoming independent. Observe this client's self-management skills. If he or she does not effectively manage cues for his or her own behavior, write a program for teaching those

skills. If he or she does not effectively manage consequences for his or her own behavior, write a program for teaching those skills. Remember that, in order to self-manage consequences, you must be able to observe your behavior, evaluate it, decide on consequences for it, and administer those consequences.

ADDITIONAL RESOURCES

Coleman, R. S., Whitman, T. L., & Johnson, M. R. Suppression of self-stimulatory behavior of a profoundly retarded boy across staff and settings: An assessment of situational generalization. *Behavior Therapy*, 1979, *10*, 266–280.

Hunter, J., & Batsone, D. A practical procedure to maintain pupils' accurate self-rating in a classroom token program. *Behavior Modification*, 1978, *2*, 93–112.

Litrownik, A. J., & Freitas, J. L. Self-monitoring in moderately retarded adolescents: Reactivity and accuracy as a function of valence. *Behavior Therapy*, 1980, *11*, 245–255.

REFERENCES

Coffman, T. L., & Harris, M. C., Jr. Transition shock and adjustments of mentally retarded persons. *Mental Retardation*, 1980, *18*, 3–7.

Connis, R. T. The effects of sequential pictorial cues, self-recording, and praise on the job task sequencing of retarded adults. *Journal of Applied Behavior Analysis*, 1979, *12*, 355–361.

Dorow, L. G. Generalization effects of newly conditioned reinforcers. *Education and Training of the Mentally Retarded*, 1980, *15*, 8–14.

Gardner, W. I. *Learning and behavior characteristics of exceptional children and youth: A humanistic behavioral approach*. Boston: Allyn & Bacon, 1977.

Hall, R. V. *Managing Behavior* (Part 2). Lawrence, Kans.: H & H Enterprises, 1975.

Holman, J. The moral risk and high cost of ecological concern in applied behavior analysis. In A. Rogers-Warren & S. F. Warren (Eds.), *Ecological perspectives in behavior analysis*. Baltimore: University Park Press, 1977.

Kazdin, A. E. *Behavior modification in applied settings*. Homewood, Ill.: Dorsey, 1975.

Langone, J., & Westling, D. L. Generalization of prevocational and vocational skills: Some practical tactics. *Education and Training of the Mentally Retarded*, 1979, *14*, 216–221.

Luthans, F., & Kreitner, R. *Organizational behavior modification*. Glenview, Ill.: Scott, Foresman, 1975.

Marholin, D., II, Siegel, L. J., & Phillips, D. Treatment and transfer: A search for empirical procedures. In M. Hersen, R. M. Eisler, & P. M. Miller (Eds.), *Progress in behavior modification* (Vol. 3). New York: Academic Press, 1976.

Martin, G., & Pear, J. *Behavior modification: What it is and how to do it*. Englewood Cliffs, N.J.: Prentice-Hall, 1978.

Neef, N. A., Iwata, B. A., & Page, T. J. Public transportation training in vivo versus classroom instruction. *Journal of Applied Behavior Analysis*, 1978, *11*, 331–344.

Nutter, D., & Reed, D. H. Teaching retarded women a clothing selection skill using community norms. *Journal of Applied Behavior Analysis*, 1978, *11*, 475–487.

O'Donnell, C. R. Behavior modification in community settings. In M. Hersen, R. M. Eisler, & P. M. Miller (Eds.), *Progress in behavior modification* (Vol. 4). New York: Academic Press, 1977.

Shapiro, E. S., & Klein, R. D. Self-management of classroom behavior with retarded/disturbed children. *Behavior Modification*, 1980, *4*, 83-97.

Stokes, T. F., & Baer, D. M. An implicit technology of generalization. *Journal of Applied Behavior Analysis*, 1977, *10*, 349-367.

Sulzer, B., & Mayer, G. R. *Behavior modification procedures for school personnel*. Hinsdale, Ill.: Dryden, 1972.

Chapter 12

The Systematic Programming Strategy

OBJECTIVES

To be able to:

1. Describe the steps in the systematic programming strategy.
2. Use the systematic programming strategy to develop behavioral programs.
3. Analyze program failures using the troubleshooting suggestions in this chapter and identify where the program development process has failed.
4. Provide possible solutions to program failures.

OVERALL PERSPECTIVES:
BEHAVIOR MANAGEMENT, BEHAVIORAL SYSTEMS, AND ECOLOGY

This chapter is devoted to describing the application of a systematic strategy for developing programs. We have found this strategy to be helpful in providing a framework for analyzing and developing solutions for client problems in a systematic fashion. However, before we describe the strategy itself and its various elements, we would like to first describe three ways of thinking about human behavior that have had a major impact on the development of the strategy. The first of these, which we have referred to throughout this text as behavior management, has also been referred to as behavior modification or behavior therapy. Although there is a considerable amount of controversy about how to define the behavioral approach to solving human problems, it is possible to identify a core set of characteristics common to all behavioral approaches (Kazdin & Hersen, 1980):

1. A strong commitment to the data-based evaluation of intervention procedures;

2. A belief that intervention must include opportunities to learn adaptive behaviors;
3. The specification of interventions in operational terms; and
4. The evaluation of intervention effects across various response measures with particular emphasis on overt observable behavior.

These characteristics form the basis for much of what you have read and worked with so far in this text. You will continue to find an emphasis on these characteristics through the remainder of this book.

The second major perspective that has influenced our thinking is known as the systems approach to behavior. This approach implies that you must view the world of behavior as composed of behavioral systems and subsystems that function as wholes (Wahler, Berland, Coe, & Leske, 1977). Furthermore, the systems approach assumes that behavioral systems function as a whole by virtue of the interdependence of their parts (Zifferblatt, 1973).

The final way of thinking about behavior that has had a strong impact on the development of this chapter is the ecological approach. Most people think of the natural environment when they hear a reference to ecology; that is, how various types of plants or animals affect each other, effects of air pollution, or how adding something to an ocean affects the animal life in it. However, we refer to behavioral ecology. More specifically, we refer to two behavioral ecologies as defined by Rogers-Warren and Warren (1977). The first ecology we refer to is the system of intrapersonal behavior. This means behavior within an individual. The notion of an intrapersonal system of behavior—that is, one that exists within a given individual—has very definite implications for how we look at the individual's behavior. The implications are that there are response clusters of behaviors that are related in some way. Furthermore, the effects of programming may well appear not only as changes in the target behavior but also as changes in related behaviors that are part of the same response cluster. O'Donnell (1977), in discussing response clusters, has observed that effects of intervention on nontargeted behaviors may be positive or negative. Negative effects may include the occurrence of new deviant behaviors when old ones are ignored, and positive effects may include increased inappropriate social skills when the target is a decrease in aggressive behaviors. The point of all of this is that no single behavior or group of behaviors exists in isolation (Gardner, 1977).

The second type of ecology we are concerned with is an interpersonal as opposed to an intrapersonal ecology. Interpersonal ecology refers not just to systems among people but also includes various aspects of the physical environment, as well as the people in it. In other words, interpersonal ecologies include buildings, furniture and how it is arranged, traffic patterns, and so forth, as well as people. In order to bring together these two types of systems, consider the approach that suggests that each individual functions on at least four different system levels. These levels are similar to the four levels described by Belsky (1980). The first level is the intraindividual system. This system consists of all of the individual's behaviors, including the relationships among them, as well as other characteristics such as physical skills or impairments that affect behavior. The second level system is the system that includes the individual and his or her immediate everyday surroundings. This system is composed of the places and people that the individual regularly encounters during his or her daily routine, such as parents, friends, group home, apartment, workshop, and school. The third system level is the larger social system that contains the individual's immediate environment. This system includes the community, the city, county, state, the legal system, the church structure, and so forth, as well as all of the people who are parts of those structures. The fourth system is the system of overriding cultural beliefs and practices in which the other three systems exist. For instance, the popular literature often makes a distinction between Eastern (meaning Asian) and Western (meaning European and American) culture. These two cultures differ in how they teach people to behave in relation to religion and concepts of honor, to give just two examples. It is also common, particularly in the United States, to find very different cultural systems operating within the same country. For example, the Native American or American Indian culture is very different from that of most other residents of this country.

Now, why is all of this important? It is important because every time we make a change in a system it is extremely likely that that change will have results either in addition to or instead of the results we want it to have (Marston, 1979). Obviously behavioral systems are extremely complex and we cannot possibly predict in advance all possible outcomes of changing a given system. However, what we can do is specify in observable terms what we have done and measure in an observable fashion the results of what we have done. We can also attempt to make our interventions change existing systems as little as possible in order to not create a whole host of unexpected side effects. Hence, the need to remember our ecological behavioral systems approach to thinking about human behavior as we proceed through the programming strategy.

SYSTEMATIC PROGRAMMING STRATEGY

Overview

At first glance the programming strategy appears very simple. It consists of the following steps:

1. Define the problem.
2. Formulate hypotheses about what is maintaining the problem.
3. Identify possible program options that will solve the problem.

4. Choose from among those options.
5. Evaluate the results of the options selected.
6a. If the program is effective, program for maintenance and generalization of the behavior change; or
6b. If the program is not effective, try to figure out why not and change the program so that it will be effective.

A diagram or flowchart laying out this strategy is shown in Figure 12-1. A worksheet we have found to be very useful during the first four steps of the strategy is shown in Figure 12-2. We will refer to this worksheet often as we discuss each individual step of the programming strategy.

Define the Problem

You will notice that on the problem worksheet there are three columns to be filled in under the problem column: Does Do, Should Do, and Classification.

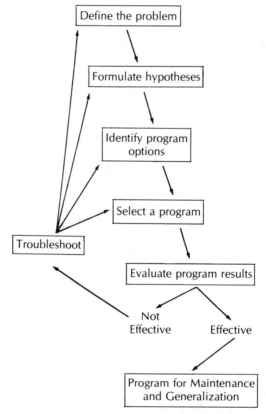

Figure 12-1. A strategy for behavior managers.

Worksheet for Behavior Problem Analysis

Client _____   Date _____   Staff Doing Analysis _____

Problem		Possible Correlates	Program Resources	Program Options	Evaluation of Options	
Does Do	Should Do (Goal) / Classification				Advantages	Disadvantages

Figure 12-2. A worksheet for behavior problem analysis.

The Does Do column should be filled in with a description of what the individual is doing at the present time. This description should be based on direct observation of behavior using one of the observation techniques discussed in Chapter 6. Should Do refers to what you want the behavior to look like after you program the changes. In other words, Should Do refers to the goal. One reason that it is absolutely critical to have a goal in mind as you go about defining and analyzing the problem is that no behavior is inherently inappropriate or inadequate. Rather, there is a discrepancy between what people do and what you expect them to do (Gardner, 1977).

The process of setting programming goals has been discussed in detail in Chapters 4 and 5. We will not, therefore, spend a great deal of time discussing goal selection. However, there are some general questions that you should probably consider as you begin to define a behavior problem. Remember that a behavior is only a problem if there is a discrepancy between what an individual does and what people expect him or her to do. Therefore, in defining a problem we must consider the expectations that people have for each other and for themselves (Laten & Wikler, 1978).

Several authors, such as Kazdin (1975), have suggested that behavior change should only be attempted if it is socially significant. One way of deciding whether a significant behavior problem exists is to ask how different the individual's current behavior is from the behavior of individuals not seen as targets for programming (O'Donnell, 1977). In addition to asking whether the individual's behavior is significantly different from other individuals who are not receiving services, it is also important to ask if this problem is important to the client or to others (Martin & Pear, 1978). Another way of asking this question is to say "Who's problem is it?" (Karan, Bernstein, Harvey, Bates, Renzaglia, & Rosenthal, 1979). You need to consider whether the individual's behavior must change in order for that individual to become an independent member of his or her community. If the answer to that question is "no," you probably shouldn't be designing a program. For example, the authors have frequently been asked to assist in the design of a program to change the behavior of clients who talk to themselves. In many cases, we have been reluctant to encourage the development of such a program because we know a great many competent individuals, including some of us, who talk to themselves. Our general guideline for making these types of decisions is that there is often not enough time to provide programming for important problems. Spending time on problems that are defined by staff idiosyncracies rather than by the demands of the community seems wasteful.

A Behavior Classification System You will notice that the third column under the problem section of the behavior problem analysis worksheet is entitled Classification. We have found that classifying the type of behavior problem with which we are dealing helps us to think about how we might solve that problem. We are not referring to classifying a problem in the sense of providing a label that implies some type of underlying cause. Instead, we are referring to a descriptive classification system that is based on the work of William Gardner (1977). The version of the classification system that we use was adapted from work by Gardner (1977) and Karan et al. (1979) and is shown in Table 12-1.

You will notice that the classification system divides behavior problems into two general categories: deficits and excesses. A deficit in behavior means that you are observing less of a desired behavior than you want to see, and an excess of behavior means that you are observing more of a particular behavior than is desired. It is extremely important that you remember that for every deficit in behavior there is a corresponding excess. Even more important, for every excess in behavior there is a corresponding deficit. When people start telling us about behavior problems, the large majority of the time they talk about excesses in behavior, that is, that they are seeing too much of an undesirable behavior. Whenever you find yourself doing this, ask instead "What is the deficit that corresponds to this excess? What do I want this person to be doing instead of what I now see them doing?" This will identify the corresponding deficit and will provide you with the means of defining your goal. It is almost always more productive to write programs that are based on

Table 12-1. Classification system for behavior excesses or deficits[a]

Deficits

A. Absence of desired behavior. Behavior of the form required does not occur on those occasions in which the correct form is expected.

B. Deficits in those behaviors necessary to meet the demands of the situation.

    1. Correct form of the behavior is present but does not consistently occur on those occasions on which it is expected.

    2. Behavior is not of the correct form (approximation only) but consistently occurs on those occasions on which the correct form is expected.

    3. Behavior is not of the correct form (approximation only) nor does it consistently occur on those occasions on which the correct form is expected.

Excesses

C. Excessive inappropriate emotional, verbal, and/or motor behavior occurs in situation(s) in which desired behavior of the correct form is absent.

D. Excessive inappropriate emotional, verbal, and/or motor behavior occurs in situation(s) in which it competes with behavior of the correct form.

E. Excessive inappropriate emotional, verbal, and/or motor behavior occurs in situation(s) in which there is sufficient behavior of the correct form.

F. Excessive inappropriate emotional, verbal, and/or motor behavior occurs to such an extent that an evaluation of appropriate behavior is not possible.

[a] Adapted from Karan, O. C., Bernstein, G. S., Harvey, J., Bates, P., Renzaglia, A., & Rosenthal, D. An extended evaluation model for severely handicapped persons. *AAESPH Review*, 1979, *4*, 374–398.

solving a behavior deficit. That is because it is a much more positive, adaptive approach to say "I want to teach this person to do more of something desirable" than "I want to teach this person to do less of something undesirable." Now let's take a look at the specific categories in the classification system.

The first category is the absence of desired behavior. Behavior of the form required does not occur on those occasions in which the correct form is expected. This means that you have never seen the individual display the desired behavior. If you have seen the individual display the desired behavior in any way at all then the problem classification is one or more of those listed under B in Table 12-1: deficits in those behaviors necessary to meet the demands of the situation. The first possibility is that the correct form of the behavior is present but does not consistently occur on those occasions on which it is expected. For instance, suppose an individual is expected to make her bed every morning. When she does make the bed it is made according to the standards for bedmaking you have set. However, she does not make the bed every morning but rather only one out of every two mornings. This is a behavior that is present in the correct form but does not consistently occur when it is supposed to. Second, behavior can be classified as not of the correct form but occurring consistently on those occasions when the correct form is expected. This might be an individual who consistently works on a five-step task whenever he is supposed to, but only completes three of the five steps. Finally, behavior can be classified as neither of the correct form nor occurring consistently when the correct form is expected. To continue the example above, this might be an individual who works on the five-step task, does not complete all five steps, and does not consistently work during scheduled work time.

There are four possible classifications for excesses in behavior. First, there are excessive inappropriate emotional, verbal, and/or motor behaviors that occur in situations where the desired behavior of the correct form is absent. This might be an individual who cries, talks to you, or wanders around the room instead of working. The second classification of excesses is excessive inappropriate emotional, verbal, and/or motor behaviors in situations where they compete with behavior of the correct form. An individual who has displayed high-quality work production at competitive rates but who occasionally becomes very angry and displays temper tantrums that interfere with his or her work would be displaying this kind of behavior excess.

The third category is excessive inappropriate emotional, verbal, and/or motor behaviors in situations in which there is sufficient behavior of the correct form. An individual who has breakfast, takes a shower, gets dressed, cleans his or her room—in short, does everything necessary to get ready to go to work—and then spends the 10 minutes between when chores are finished and when he or she is supposed to leave for work harassing another resident is displaying this type of excess. The final type of excess in this classification system is excessive inappropriate behavior to such an extent that evaluation of appropriate behavior is not possible. In thinking about the different kinds of excessive behavior problems, once again you must remember to be very careful in how you use the word appropriate or inappropriate. Remember, a behavior is only appropriate or inappropriate in relation to somebody's standards for what the behavior should look like and when and where the behavior should occur. Make very sure when you label a behavior inappropriate that you know what standards you are referring to, who determined them, and whether they are in fact important in terms of the client's overall goals.

In identifying the three items that come under the Problem section of the worksheet, Does Do, Should Do, and Classification, you will often find yourself rewriting the Does Do and/or the Goals as you look at the classification. There is no one set order in which these three things should come. Rather, these items are very interactive, and as you begin to classify a behavior you may find yourself wanting to look at it in a different way. Obviously you will have to start with a problem statement of some sort in the Does Do category. However, there is nothing wrong with redefining your problem as you go through this analysis. Once you have defined your problem the next step in the program strategy is to identify some possible correlates that may be maintaining the problem situation.

Identify Possible Correlates of the Behavior

When two events or variables are related in some systematic way we say that they are correlates of each other or that the two events are correlated. The approach we are taking to client programming suggests that we examine the environment to identify possible correlates of behavior problems in order for us to be able to identify what we want to change about the environment. We say correlate and not cause because there is no way to ever be sure what is causing a behavior without going back and creating a situation that then results in the behavior we think it caused. This is extremely impractical, usually unethical, and not really necessary. The reason that it is not really necessary is that very often the factors that are influencing or maintaining a behavior in the present may not have been involved at all or not involved to the same extent in the original development of the behavior (Gardner, 1977). Thus, it is really not important what originally caused a behavior pattern to develop. What is important is what is maintaining the behavior in the present, because that is what has to be changed in order to change the behavior.

As we go through the process of identifying possible correlates you may wonder why we just don't have a checklist of correlates for each type of behavior problem that can be applied in general. The reason we do not have such a list is that, although a behavior may appear to be very similar in two different people, the factors influencing that behavior may in fact be very different (Gardner, 1977). Also, there are times that two different behavior patterns that appear to have nothing to do with each other in two different people are in fact being maintained by the same factors. Hence, the need to individually analyze possible correlates of behavior problems for each individual.

Table 12-2 lists some typical correlates of behavior excesses or deficits. The first correlate and the one that should always be considered is that the target behavior is not in the individual's repertoire. When we are consulted about developing programs for clients we are often told so and so *won't* do whatever the desired behavior is. Our immediate response is going to be, have you ever seen this person perform this behavior? If the answer to that question is "no," then it is not that the individual won't do it, it's that the individual

Table 12-2. Possible correlates of behavior deficits or excesses[a]

 I. Target behavior not in individual's repertoire.
 II. Antecedent events difficulties
   A. Relevant cues too restricted in number or type
   B. Relevant cues not available
   C. Irrelevant cues interfere with recognition of relevant cues
   D. Emotional arousal interferes with recognition of cues.
   E. Inappropriate cues available in environment
   F. Occurrence of internal cues for inappropriate behavior
   G. Training cues not sufficiently similar to naturally occurring cues
 III. Consequence difficulties
   A. Environment not sufficiently reinforcing
     1. Source of reinforcement unreliable
     2. Schedule inadequate
     3. Too few sources of reinforcement
       A. External
       B. Internal
   B. Competing behaviors reinforced
     1. Naturally occurring reinforcers more powerful than those available from training environment
     2. Self-reinforcement of competing behaviors.
   C. Inappropriate use of punishment
     1. Too many or too severe aversive consequences relative to available reinforcement
     2. Inappropriate self-punishment
     3. Individual does not have acceptable alternative behavior in repertoire

[a] Adapted from Karan, O. C., Bernstein, G. S., Harvey, J., Bates, P., Renzaglia, A., & Rosenthal, D. An extended evaluation model for severely handicapped persons. *AAESPH Review*, 1979, *4*, 374–398.

has never learned how. This is a much more positive way of looking at the problem. If someone doesn't know how to do something you can then proceed to teach them what to do, whereas if you assume that they are refusing to do something they have already learned you have a negative situation.

The next main category of possible correlates has to do with difficulties related to antecedent events. Antecedent events occur just before a behavior is supposed to occur. We have identified seven possible difficulties with antecedents. The first is that relevant cues may be too restricted in number or type. For example, some people are such heavy sleepers that they need two or three alarm clocks that go off at set intervals in order to get out of bed in the morning. If one of those individuals is given only one alarm clock, the odds are pretty good that, because the relevant cues are too restricted, they are not going to make it out of bed on time. The second type of difficulty with antecedent events is that the relevant cues are not available. This would be a case where there was no alarm clock available that a heavy sleeper could use. A third possibility is that the appropriate number and type of relevant cues are available but irrelevant cues interfere with the recognition of the relevant ones. Anyone who has ever shut off an alarm clock because the phone was ringing knows how an irrelevant cue can interfere with recognition of relevant ones.

Next, emotional arousal can interfere with the recognition of cues. If you are extremely upset about something you are probably going to pay a lot less attention to cues that normally cue you to start a particular task. This is an important point because it implies that, when one of the people you serve is extremely upset, that is not the time to force a confrontation about whether they attend to normal cues such as instructions to go back to work. The next category is the availability of inappropriate cues in the environment. If you ever were or had a class with a typical class clown you know what this one is all about. Usually the class clown gets going because other members of the class start asking for a favorite routine. This is a case of inappropriate cues being available in the environment (at least inappropriate in the teacher's opinion).

Also it is possible for internal cues for inappropriate behavior to occur. Many people occasionally go through an internal process where, after making a minor mistake, they think "I'm not doing the job right. They must think I'm not doing a good job. They must think I'm an awful person." The next thing you know you have got yourself so upset that you can't do anything. This is a case of cuing yourself for inappropriate behavior—that is to say, nonproductive behavior. The difficulty, of course, with identifying this kind of possible correlate is that you have to get the client to verbalize whatever internal cues he or she is providing in order to identify them as possible correlates.

The last type of antecedent event difficulty is the situation where training cues are not sufficiently similar to naturally occurring cues. Let's take a look at just one example. In early training programs developmentally disabled individuals were often taught to identify the correct public restroom by learning to distinguish between signs that said "men" and "women." Unfortunately, the naturally occurring cues for discriminating between men's and women's restrooms in public places are often not very similar to those training cues. There may be signs that say "cowboys" and "cowgirls" or "dukes" and "duchesses" or "ladies" and "gentlemen," there may not be words at all but rather just pictures, or there may be words in a language other than English. All of these represent situations where the naturally occurring cues are not very similar at all to the training cues.

The third category of possible correlates of behavior problems refers to difficulties with consequences. One of the most common programming failures is the failure to provide an environment that is sufficiently reinforcing for desired behaviors. This may be for one of three reasons. First, the source of reinforcement may be unreliable. If you provide a lot of verbal praise one day and very little the next because you are not feeling well, then you are an unreliable source of reinforcement. The second possibility is that the schedule of reinforcement is inadequate. Remember in Chapter 11 we discussed the need to thin schedules of reinforcement gradually. If you thin out the available reinforcement too quickly and the behavior starts to drop off, you have an inadequate schedule of reinforcement. The environment may not be providing enough sources of reinforcement. An example of too few sources of reinforcement in the external environment might be that you've got only one staff person reinforcing a behavior when two or three are needed. The question of internal sources of reinforcement relates to the whole issue of self-management. If an individual is unable to provide sufficient self-reinforcement, he or she will be unable to maintain his or her behavior.

The second type of difficulty with consequences is that behaviors that compete with desired behaviors may be reinforced, either by self-reinforcement or by naturally occurring reinforcers. The class clown's behavior is often reinforced by attention from peers. Peer attention is often more powerful than the reinforcers provided by the teacher. Alternatively, the class clown may be maintained by self-reinforcement. That is, the clown is telling himself or herself "I'm a wonderful person because I make everybody laugh."

The final type of consequence difficulty that we often encounter is the inappropriate use of punishment. There are at least three possible ways in which punishment can be used inappropriately. First, there may be too many consequences or consequences that are too severe relative to available reinforcement. Depriving someone of their dessert, sending them to bed early, and banning them from a group outing the following week is a combination of aversive consequences that is probably too severe for someone who has failed to come to the dinner table on time. Similarly, locking someone in isolation for several hours at a time is too severe, particularly when you are locking them away from an environment where there is relatively little reinforcement available. The second type of inappropriate use of punishment is inappropriate self-punishment. This relates back to our description of people who tell themselves what terrible people they are because they made one small mistake. The final type of inappropriate use of punishment is the use of punishment when individuals do not have acceptable alternative behaviors in their repertoires. This classification is very closely related to the first correlate we discussed: the target behavior is not in the individual's repertoire. It is not appropriate to punish someone for expressing their anger by screaming and shouting if they have never learned an acceptable alternative means of expressing anger. It is much more appropriate to teach them an alternative means of expressing anger.

There are two general things that must be kept in mind as you try to identify what you think are the possible correlates of a particular behavior problem. The first is that very often there is more than one correlate of a given behavior problem. For instance, there may be too many irrelevant cues available for competing behaviors and there may also be insufficient sources of reinforcement. So, don't stop just because you think you have identified one possible correlate. Go through the list and make sure you have covered what appear to be all of the options. The second thing to keep in mind is that, as you fill out a problem analysis worksheet and identify possible correlates, don't forget that they are *possible* correlates. What you have done is made an educated guess about what is related to the behavior problem based on your observation of the individual in his or her environment. Until you have chosen a program that is based on your possible correlates and implemented that program, you will not know whether the correlates you have identified are anything more than guesses.

Client Characteristics as Possible Correlates   The major thrust of this book has been away from the idea that the client's problems reside within the client. However, there are certain client characteristics that must be considered during a systematic approach to program development. We need to know whether the individual has any physical limitations, whether there is any sensory impairment, whether there is any evidence for neurological impairment, whether there are any particular health problems, and so forth. We particularly need to know whether the client is on any medication and if so which medications, how much of each, and whether there have been any changes in them recently. The reason we need to know about these things is because physical characteristics do affect behavior, and there is no point in developing a behavioral program for a problem that lends itself to a medical solution.

There are also some basic characteristics such as age, sex, and previous living history that will have some impact on the types of goals that are chosen for a particular individual. Clearly, the same types of work loads may not be chosen for a 57-year-old man as for a 17-year-old man. It is also important to identify the cultural background from which the client comes, particularly if it is one that is likely to be noticeably different from the cultural background of most other clients and staff. An example of this would be a client who comes from a black inner-city ghetto who is placed in a sheltered workshop in a white middle-class neighborhood. Finally, we must consider client learning histories and current skill levels when designing programs. Programs often fail because they are based on faulty assumptions about what clients can already do. Table 12-3 provides a list of considerations for matching programs to client characteristics.

Identify Program Options

The last section of the worksheet for behavior problem analysis, which deals with selecting a program, begins with a column for describing Program Resources. Availability of resources can affect which program option is chosen. Too often we have a tendency to think that our only resources are staff time and attention. This is why it is very helpful to list these resources, as well as any others that might potentially be useful in program design. Client characteristics, particularly client strengths, should be thought of as program resources. Other resources might include people, places, things, or anything else you can think of that might be useful for programming. A more extended discussion of possible resources in terms of other professionals and your community is to be found in Chapter 17. The important thing to remember about this column is to be creative. There is no set restricted list of program resources.

The next column on the problem analysis worksheet is for identifying Possible Program Options. Program options are simply specific applications of the types of procedures described in Chapters 8 through 11. A quick summary list of them is shown in Table 12-4. Remember, however, that it is not sufficient to simply list positive reinforcement or timeout under Program Options. Instead, indicate how positive reinforcement or timeout will be used in relation to the particular behavior problem that is being analyzed.

Select a Program Option

The last two columns on the problem analysis worksheet are for listing the advantages and disadvantages of each program option. The three types of advantages and disadvantages that should be considered for each option relate to three questions:

1. Does the option make sense?
2. Is it practical?
3. It is legal and ethical?

Table 12-3. Checklist for matching program to client characteristics[a]

When Designing	Consider
Antecedents	
Auditory cues	
1. Verbal	Vocabulary
	Length of statements
	Complexity of statements
	Volume
	Tone
2. Other	Competing noises
	Bell vs. buzzer vs. clap vs. etc.
Visual cues	
1. Social	Eye contact
	Facial gestures
	Body gestures
	Physical contact
2. Tangible	Number of cues
	Redundancy
	Relevance
	Proximity
	Color
	Size
	Shape
	Complexity
	Novelty
	Type (e.g., jig, counter)
General contextual cues	
1. Setting	Seating arrangements
	Task
	Visual distractions
	Auditory distractions
2. Policy	Rules for clients
	Staff expectations
	Consistency level
3. Social	Peer behavior
	Staff as models
Consequences	Density of schedule
	Length of delay
	Method of delivery
	Natural vs. artificial
	Cues or reminders

[a] Adapted from K. Tyser (personal communication, 1976).

Table 12–4. Intervention strategies

Teaching Strategies

Task analysis	Fading
Instructions	Chaining
Modeling/imitation	Positive practice
Prompting	Role-playing
Shaping	

Use of Antecedents

Instructions	Remove irrelevant cues
Modeling—staff, peer	Remove cues for inappropriate behaviors
Prompting—physical	Behavioral contracting
Add cues for appropriate behavior	Teach self-cuing
Add more relevant cues	

Use of Consequences

Increasing occurrence of behavior

1. Type of reinforcer (value)
   Edible
   Tangible
   Social
   Premack
   Naturally occurring
   Generalized

2. Schedule of reinforcement
   Variable vs. fixed
   Interval vs. ratio
   Delayed vs. immediate
3. Reinforcer sampling
4. Self-control
   Self-monitoring
   Self-evaluation
   Self-reinforcement

Decreasing occurrence of behavior

1. Reinforcing alternative behaviors
2. DRO
3. Extinction

4. Timeout
5. Response cost
6. Overcorrection

Go back and ask yourself if you and the people you work with are the appropriate people to deal with this problem (Martin & Pear, 1978). For instance, have you eliminated the possibility that the problem is caused by medical complications that should be referred to a specialist? If you are satisfied that you are the appropriate person to be dealing with this problem, then you need to ask yourself whether each program option makes sense in light of your problem analysis. If the problem has been classified as a deficit, is your program designed to increase a behavior or teach a new behavior? If the problem is an excess, is your program designed to decrease the excess? You also need to consider whether your program options make sense in light of the possible correlates that you have listed. If a lack of relevant cues for the desired behavior in the environment is one of your possible correlates, does your program arrange for the provision of additional cues? If one of your possible correlates is inconsistent sources of reinforcement, does your program arrange to make sources of reinforcement more consistent?

The next type of advantage or disadvantage to be considered is whether each of your program options is practical. Some of the considerations under this type of advantage or disadvantage include whether the people in your setting are willing to implement this option, whether they possess the skills necessary to collect data on the behavior, and whether they have the time and the resources to implement the options (Karan et al., 1979). Considerations here also include whether you have adequate control of the contingencies so that you are able to manipulate them (Sulzer & Mayer, 1972) and, if there are hindrances to implementing a particular option, whether you have ways to minimize the effects of those hindrances (Martin & Pear, 1978).

The final type of advantage or disadvantage that must be considered as you weigh the merits of various program options has to do with whether you have chosen a program that meets both legal and ethical standards. For each program option you need to consider:

1. Whether the goal has been chosen for the client's benefit (Martin & Pear, 1978).
2. Whether the specific goal is related to long-term goals for this individual (Gardner, 1977).
3. Whether all legal requirements for designing client programs have been met.
4. Whether you have chosen the least intrusive method possible that is likely to be effective for changing the particular behavior of interest.
5. Whether you have preserved all legally determined client rights such as the right to a balanced diet and a certain amount of privacy. Since legal regulations relating to client rights and what is considered legal programming change over time, and vary from state to state and among different types of programs, it is suggested that you become familiar with the laws and regulations governing client programming in your facility and in your state.

Write the Program

Once you have selected a program option it is time to write the complete program. A good behavior management program is written in enough detail so that you can tell from reading it what behavior is being changed, what it is being changed to, and why it is being changed. It will then tell you where the program is to occur, when, with what, who is going to do it, what they are going to do, and how they are going to do it. Finally, a good program will tell you how program results are going to be evaluated, who is going to be responsible for evaluating them, how data are going to be collected, and how

Program Form

Client _____

Date Program Begins _____

I. Behavior
    A. Target behavior _____

        _____

    B. Current behavior _____

        _____

    C. Why program is needed _____

        _____

        _____

II. Conditions
    A. Where? (location) _____

        _____

    B. When? (schedule) _____

        _____

    C. With what? (materials) _____

        _____

    D. By whom? (people responsible) _____

        _____

III. Method
    A. What to do and how to do it
        1. Before behavior occurs (antecedents) _____

            _____

            _____

        2. After behavior occurs (consequences and contingencies) _____

            _____

            _____

IV. Evaluation
    A. Attach completed Measurement Procedure Form
    B. Who is responsible for regular review of the data? _____

        _____

    C. When are these reviews to occur? _____

        _____

        _____

Figure 12-3.   Sample program form.

often reviews of results are going to occur. It will be much easier to write a good program if you use a standard form that requires you to fill in all of this information. One possible form is shown in Figure 12-3.

Once the program has been written it is helpful to go back and review questions about possible advantages and disadvantages of this particular program to make sure that this still appears to be the best possible choice. So, take the completed program and once again ask yourself: does this program make sense, is it practical, and does it meet legal and ethical standards?

Evaluate Program Results

If regular reviews of the data indicate that your program has been effective, the next step is to program for maintenance and generalization of the behavior change. Techniques for programming for maintenance and generalization were discussed in detail in Chapter 11. The elements of a good program for maintenance and generalization are exactly the same as the elements of any other good behavior management program and a form similar to the one shown in Figure 12-3 is recommended as a basis for writing such programs.

TROUBLESHOOTING

What do you do if at regular evaluations of your data you find that your program is not effective? Well, it's obviously time to do some troubleshooting. Before looking at any of the possibilities for changing a program, the first question you need to ask yourself is whether the program has really been used as written (Deno & Mirkin, 1980). In other words, you need to take a look at whether the program that you designed was in fact implemented the way it was supposed to be. If not, then maybe the problem is not with the program but with the way it's being used. This type of problem occurs either because the program is too complex to be practical or because the people who are supposed to use it do not agree with program design. If the problem is lack of staff agreement, maybe staff have not been involved enough in program design.

Now, if the program has been used the way it was planned, then what? If you look back at Figure 12-1, the flow chart that lays out the strategy for behavior managers, you will notice that when the program is not effective the lines for troubleshooting go back to any one of the steps in the strategy process. This is because the problem with the program could be at any one of these steps. At the problem definition step, two possible difficulties are that the goal that has been selected is too difficult or that there are too many goals (Karan et al., 1979). At the formulate-the-hypotheses stage, maybe the possible correlates are incorrect or maybe you haven't identified all of them. For example, there may be other events occurring during program intervention that are influencing the client's behavior or there may be aversive events that result in the individual avoiding the programming situation (Karan et al., 1979). Perhaps the goal and the possible correlates are logical but there is a flaw in the program. For instance, the prompts used may not be appropriate for the client's level of functioning, the consequences may not be presented frequently enough, or consequences may not be presented promptly enough (Karan et al., 1979). Sometimes, although not very often, progress is occurring but the procedure for collecting data on client progress has not been designed in a way that reflects small behavior changes.

Human behavior is so complex that your programs will often require revision, sometimes many revisions. When you have reached the point where you can't think of another way of changing the program that might be helpful, it is time to call in outside help. All of the authors have spent a considerable amount of time as outside consultants who are called in for assistance when programs aren't working. We find that we are successful in suggesting effective programming strategies not just because we are experts in behavioral programming, although that is the necessary condition. Rather, it is the combination of having behavioral skills and having a different, outside perspective that makes us effective as consultants. In other words, sometimes when you are in the middle of a situation it is difficult to see the forest for the trees and therefore easy to miss some key factor that is making a program ineffective. An outside perspective can help you find the forest again.

AN EXAMPLE OF SYSTEMATIC PROGRAMMING

This section is designed to show you how the systematic programming strategy can be used. The client and staff are not real, but the problem and its solution are similar to many real situations we have encountered.

Defining the Problem

Ron Vocational Trainer comes to Sally Behavior Manager for help with one of his clients, Joan Brown. He's begun to analyze the problem, and the first section of his worksheet looks like this:

Client: _Joan Brown_____

Problem		
Does Do	Should Do (Goal)	Classification
Wanders around room, flaps hands, sometimes on task, touches male staff	Not wander, flap, or touch male staff	Excess—excessive motor behavior competes with behavior of correct form

Sally suggests that it will probably be more helpful to think of the problem as a deficit rather than an excess. She recommends they start with a worksheet that begins:

Client: _Joan Brown_

Problem		
Does Do	Should Do (Goal)	Classification
Wanders around room, flaps hands, sometimes on task, touches male staff	Work on-task 100% of time during 10:30– 12:00 work period	Deficit—behavior of correct form does not consistently occur when expected

Ron agrees this is a more helpful approach. He also suggests that, while they work on the analysis, he begin collecting baseline data on Joan's on-task behavior. Sally agrees, and they design the measurement procedure shown in Figure 12-4 (pages 236–237).

Formulating Hypotheses

Ron and Sally now proceed with their problem analysis. To help them identify possible correlates, they examine the anecdotal records Ron has been collecting for the last week. One of these is shown in Figure 12-5. After discussing these records, they add to their worksheet so that it looks like this:

Client: _Joan Brown_   Date: _October 10, 1980_

Problem			Possible Correlates
Does Do	Should Do (Goal)	Classification	
Wanders around room, flaps hands, sometimes on task, touches male staff	Work on task 100% of time during 10:30– 12:00 work period	Deficit— behavior of correct form does not consistently occur when expected	Irrelevant cues (such as men entering room) interfere with relevant cues. Relevant cues too restricted. Schedules of reinforcement inadequate. Competing behaviors (wandering, hand flapping) being reinforced

Identifying Program Options

Sally and Ron then brainstorm a list of program resources and options. They list potential advantages and disadvantages of each option to complete their analysis, which is shown in Figure 12-6.

Measurement Procedure Form

1. Person to be observed   _Joan Brown_

2. Operational definition of behavior to be observed
   On task, which means sitting in seat at work station with at least one hand touching assigned task.

3. Dimensions of behavior to be observed   _Duration_

4. When to observe
   a. Days of week   _Mon., Tues., Wed., Thurs., Fri._
   b. Time of day   _10:45 AM –10:50 AM, 11:30 AM –11:35 AM_
   c. Dates   _Start Oct. 13, continue till notified otherwise_

5. Who observes   _Ron Vocational Trainer_

6. Where to observe   _In activity center vocational training room_

7. Tools needed
   a. Data sheet—attach to form
   b. Other—include location of each item   _Audible timer with earplug—in desk in vocational training room_

8. How to record   _Set times for 15 second intervals and put on earplug. Each time tone is heard, put + on data form if Joan is on task as defined above, – if she is not on task._

9. Graph—attach to form

10. Procedures for assessing interobserver agreement
    Sally Behavior Manager will observe at the same times as Ron one day per week.

11. Procedures for minimizing reactivity
    Ron uses record forms and the timer several times a day, so reactivity shouldn't be a big problem.

12. Procedures for training observers
    Ron and Sally have already been trained to use interval recording.

Figure 12-4.   Measurement procedure and behavior observation (interval recording) forms for Joan Brown.

Behavior Observation Form—Interval Recording

Behavior ___On task—see definition on Measurement Procedure Form___
Client __Joan Brown__ Observer ___Ron Vocational Trainer_ Date _____
Location _____
Length of intervals = __15__ seconds
Time started _____

Figure 12-4. (*continued*)

Anecdotal Record Form

Client _Joan Brown_____ Observer _Ron Vocational Trainer_Date _Oct. 7, 1980_

Time	Antecedents	Behavior	Consequences	Location
10:30 AM	I come into training room to begin work sessions	Joan walks over and starts rubbing my shoulder	I take Joan back to her work station and tell her to go to work	Training room
10:45	I look around the room.	Joan is working.	I say, "Good job, Joan –keep working."	Training room
10:55	?	Joan leaves her work station, wanders around the room flapping her hands.	Two other workers yell at Joan for disturbing them. I take her back to work.	Training room
11:05	I look around the room.	Joan is working.	I go to her and say, "You're doing well today."	Training room
11:20	Bill Administrator comes in to ask me a question.	Joan walks up to Bill and rubs his back.	He smiles, says "Hi, Joan. Are you working hard?" I take Joan back to work.	Training room

Figure 12-5. Anecdotal record form for Joan Brown's behavior.

Selecting a Program

After the worksheet is completed, Sally and Ron review the various program options and the advantages and disadvantages of each option. They decide that increasing the frequency of reinforcement for on-task behavior is the most positive option for the vocational training setting. They do, however, arrange to discuss a possible social skills training program with staff at the group home where Joan lives.

Writing the Program

The program Sally and Ron write is shown in Figure 12-7.

Worksheet for Behavior Problem Analysis

Client _Joan Brown_   Date _October 10, 1980_   Staff Doing Analysis _Ron Vocational Trainer & Sally Behavior Manager_

Problem					Evaluation of Options	
Does Do	Should Do (Goal)	Classification	Possible Correlates	Program Resources	Program Options	Advantages	Disadvantages
Wanders around room, flaps hands, sometimes on task, touches male staff	Work on task 100% of time during 10:30 – 12:00 work period	Deficit— behavior of correct form does not consistently occur when expected	Irrelevant cues (such as men entering room) interfere with relevant cues	Responds well to praise	Add cues for being on task, such as timer	Could lead to self-management by teaching her to use timer	Could be intrusive, may not help if reinforcement is insufficient
			Relevant cues too restricted	Staff ratio of 1 to 5			
			Schedule of reinforcement is inadequate	Joan is usually very cooperative, has good receptive and expressive language, has expressed desire to work hard	Transfer to female trainer	Will probably eliminate at least part of problem	Avoids problem, does not teach alternative behavior
			Competing behaviors (wandering, hand flapping) being reinforced		Do not allow other staff to enter room during training	Same as above	Same as above

(continued)

239

Worksheet for Behavior Problem Analysis (continued)

Problem			Possible Correlates	Program Resources	Program Options	Evaluation of Options	
Does Do	Should Do (Goal)	Classification				Advantages	Disadvantages
			The excessive behaviors are reported to have a long history of occurrence with no consistent programming designed to change them during Joan's 10 years in the state institution	and have dates (is 17 years old)	Increase density of reinforcement for on task	Proactive, encourage the behaviors being taught	Requires more staff attention
					Reprimand for wandering	Easy to use	Does not teach alternative. Attention of reprimand may be reinforcing
					Teach acceptable social skills for interacting with men	Proactive, teaches alternative	Social skills are not supposed to be emphasized during work training

Figure 12-6. Worksheet for behavior problem analysis for Joan Brown.

Program Form

Client __Joan Brown__

Date Program Begins ___October 20, 1980___

 I. Behavior
   A. Target behavior __On task 100% of observed intervals for 10__
       __consecutive work days__

   B. Current behavior __On task average 40% of observed intervals__

   C. Why program is needed __Increased time on task will (a) increase__
       __vocational skills and (b) be incompatible with unacceptable behaviors__
       __such as wandering, therefore increasing Joan's chance for becoming__
       __independent.__

 II. Conditions
   A. Where? (location) __Vocational training room__

   B. When? (schedule) ___10:30 AM -noon, Mon. through Fri.___

   C. With what? (materials) __None (except data form—data collection__
       __continues as during baseline)__

   D. By whom? (people responsible) __Ron Vocational Trainer__

III. Method
   A. What to do and how to do it
       1. Before behavior occurs (antecedents)
           __At 10:30, if Joan is not on task, tell her it's time to get to work__

       2. After behavior occurs (consequences and contingencies)
           __Observe Joan once during each 10-minute period from 10:30 -noon.__
           __If she is on task, walk over to her work station and praise her for__
           __working. If she is not on task, tell her to get back to work.__

IV. Evaluation
   A. Attach completed Measurement Procedure Form
   B. Who is responsible for regular review of the data? __Ron Vocational__
       __Trainer__

   C. When are these reviews to occur? __Every Friday afternoon__

Figure 12-7. Program for Joan Brown.

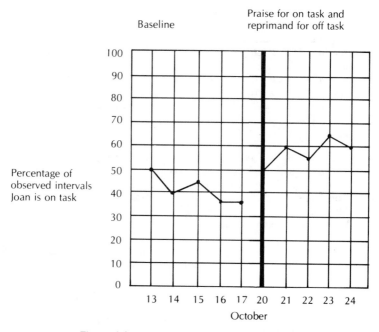

Figure 12-8.   Initial graph of Joan's on-task behavior.

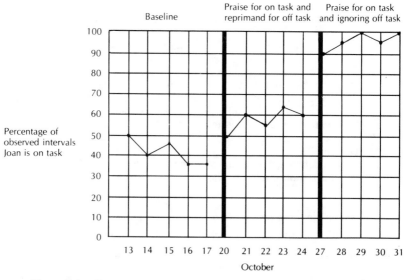

Figure 12-9.   Graph of Joan's on-task behavior after a change in reinforcement.

Evaluating Program Results

When Ron reviews the data for the first week the program was in effect, he is looking at the graph shown in Figure 12-8. He and Sally discuss the graph and agree that the increase in on-task behavior is rather small. They decide to make one change in the program. Ron will continue to praise Joan as scheduled, but will no longer tell her to get back to work when she is off task. Instead, he will ignore her when she is off task. This change is made because Ron feels that his reprimands may be reinforcing Joan for off-task behavior.

When Ron reviews the data at the end of the week, he is looking at the graph in Figure 12-9. The new program appears to be working! He and Sally decide to continue the program as is and see if Joan meets her goal under the program conditions. If she does, they will plan a program for maintaining Joan's on-task behavior.

SUGGESTED ACTIVITIES

1. The next time you need to write a program for a client, use the Worksheet for Behavior Problem Analysis. Once you have completed the Worksheet, write the complete program using the form in Figure 12-3. Did the Worksheet help you to write a good program? Why or why not? Did the Program Form help you to write a good program? Why or why not?
2. The next time you implement a program that does not succeed, look at the suggestions on troubleshooting in this chapter. Try using these suggestions to help you identify possible reasons that the program did not succeed. Use the reasons you identify to help you alter the program.

ADDITIONAL RESOURCES

These books are some of the best available descriptions of the state of the art in providing behavioral habilitation.

Bellamy, G. T., Horner, R., & Inman, D. P. *Vocational habilitation of severely retarded adults.* Baltimore: University Park Press, 1978.

Gardner, W. I. *Behavior modification in mental retardation.* Chicago: Aldine, 1971.

Gardner, W. I. *Children with learning and behavior problems.* Boston: Allyn & Bacon, 1978.

Rosen, M., Clark, G. R., & Kivitz, M. S. *Habilitation of the handicapped.* Baltimore: University Park Press, 1977.

Rusch, F. R., & Mithaug, D. E. *Vocational training for mentally retarded adults.* Champaign, Ill.: Research Press, 1980.

Sulzer-Azaroff, B., & Mayer, G. R. *Applying behavior analysis procedures with children and youth.* New York: Holt, Rinehart & Winston, 1977.

REFERENCES

Belsky, J. Child maltreatment: An ecological integration. *American Psychologist,* 1980, *35,* 320–335.

Deno, S. L., & Mirkin, P. K. Data based IEP development: An approach to substantive compliance. *Teaching Exceptional Children,* 1980, *12,* 92–97.
Gardner, W. I. *Learning and behavior characteristics of exceptional children and youth: A humanistic behavioral approach.* Boston: Allyn & Bacon, 1977.
Karan, O. C., Bernstein, G. S., Harvey, J., Bates, P., Renzaglia, A., & Rosenthal, D. An extended evaluation model for severely handicapped persons. *AAESPH Review,* 1979, *4,* 374–398.
Kazdin, A. E. *Behavior modification in applied settings.* Homewood, Ill.: Dorsey, 1975.
Kazdin, A. E., & Hersen, M. The current status of behavior therapy. *Behavior Modification,* 1980, *4,* 283–302.
Laten, S. M., & Wikler, L. *Behavioral social work assessment and intervention with families of the retarded.* Presented at the meeting of the Midwestern Association for Behavior Analysis, Chicago, 1978.
Marston, A. R. Behavior ecology emerges from behavior modification: Side-steps toward a nonspecific profession. *Behavior Modification,* 1979, *3,* 147–160.
Martin, G., & Pear, J. *Behavior modification: What it is and how to do it.* Englewood Cliffs, N.J.: Prentice-Hall, 1978.
O'Donnell, C. R. Behavior modification in community settings. In M. Hersen, R. M. Eisler, & P. M. Miller (Eds.), *Progress in behavior modification* (Vol. 4). New York: Academic Press, 1977.
Rogers-Warren, A., & Warren, S. F. The developing ecobehavioral psychology. In A. Rogers-Warren & S. F. Warren (Eds.), *Ecological perspectives in behavior analysis.* Baltimore: University Park Press, 1977.
Sulzer, B., & Mayer, R. G. *Behavior modification procedures for school personnel.* Hinsdale, Ill.: Dryden, 1972.
Wahler, R. G., Berland, R. M., Coe, T. D., & Leske, G. Social systems analysis, In A. Rogers-Warren & S. F. Warren (Eds.), *Ecological perspectives in behavior analysis.* Baltimore: University Park Press, 1977.
Zifferblatt, S. M. Behavior systems. In C. E. Thoresen (Ed.), *Behavior modification in education* (Part I). Chicago: University of Chicago Press, 1973.

Unit V

Instructional Materials
Helping Us Get There

Chapter 13

Evaluation, Adaptation, and Design of Instructional Materials

---

OBJECTIVES

To be able to:
1. Evaluate the usefulness of published instructional materials.
2. Adapt published instructional materials to fit your clients' needs.
3. Identify questions that must be considered when designing your own instructional materials.

EVALUATING INSTRUCTIONAL MATERIALS

Instructional materials are resources that should be utilized in the planning and development of habilitation programs. Currently, a wide variety of materials are available for use with developmentally disabled individuals in areas including, but not limited to, social skills, vocational skills, independent living skills, and leisure skills. The formats of these resources are varied, ranging from traditional texts to elaborate computer-based programs. Service providers should take advantage of these resources when developing client habilitation programs. Although we are certainly not advocating a cookbook approach to programming, we do encourage the application of a systematic approach to adapting materials to meet client needs. This is often less time consuming than designing your own materials. The effectiveness and utility of instructional materials, however, is still contingent upon the programming skills of the trainer (Stowitschek, Gable, & Hendrickson, 1980). Therefore, when selecting materials the focus should be both on client needs and on trainer skills.

A Checklist for Evaluating Materials[1]

The purpose of this chapter is to provide guidelines with which to select, adapt, and evaluate the effectiveness of programming materials. The checklist shown in Table 13-1 is included to assist you in evaluating materials. The checklist contains a list of questions that should be considered prior to the selection of instructional materials. It is divided into the following sections: Matching the Curriculum to Client Needs, Client Entry Skills, Structure of the Curriculum, Data Collection and Progress Assessment, Maintenance of Acquired Skills, Validation of the Curriculum, and Practical Considerations.

Matching the Curriculum to Client Needs   Initially you need to determine how appropriate the overall goals of the curriculum are for your clients. Are the goals and objectives of the curriculum consistent with your clients' goals and objectives? A one-to-one match is not necessary; however, enough of a given curriculum should be of use to your clients to make its use worth your time and effort.

Client Entry Skills   The second section of the checklist relates to the logical or developmental sequence of the curriculum and where to place clients in the sequences. For example, will acquisition of the curriculum's short-term objectives lead to the meeting of the long-term goals? This continuity between short-term objectives and long-term goals is important in the smooth progression of a client through the curriculum. The lack of such continuity within a curriculum can hinder the client's development. For example, it makes little sense to teach people to throw a ball before they have acquired the skills to grasp and hold the ball correctly. Therefore, it is imperative that the curriculum be designed logically and developmentally to accommodate the needs of the client. When appropriate, the short-term objectives should include a task analysis of the particular skill to be acquired.

The curriculum should also make provisions for assessing the client's present skill level within any particular domain. Obviously, this is extremely important for appropriate placement within the developmental sequence of the curriculum. Such appropriate placement decreases the probability that the trainer will spend useless time teaching skills that the learner already possesses or teaching skills beyond his or her current capabilities.

Structure of the Curriculum   The curriculum should provide specific instructions on how it should be implemented. For example:

---

[1]The checklist and this section of Chapter 13 were adapted from Czajkowski, L., Zawitkowski, A, & Pearce, L. *Directions in adapted physical education*. Vermillion, S.D.: Center for the Developmentally Disabled, University of South Dakota, 1980.

Table 13-1. Checklist for evaluating instructional materi

Evaluation Item		
A. Match the Curriculum to Client Needs		
Do the goals and objectives of the curriculum meet your clients' needs as indicated by their long-term goals and short-term objectives?	Yes	No
B. Client Entry Skills		
1. Does the curriculum have specifically stated long-term goals?	Yes	No
2. Does the curriculum specifically state short-term objectives?	Yes	No
3. Are the short-term objectives task analyzed within the curriculum?	Yes	No
4. Within the curriculum, do the short-term objectives provide functional task analysis of the long-term goals?	Yes	No
5. Does the curriculum make provisions for assessing the client's skills across the relevant domains? (acquisition of baseline data)	Yes	No
6. Does the curriculum specify prerequisite language skills (receptive and/or expressive) needed by the client for entry into the curriculum?	Yes	No
7. Are specific prerequisite skills for each short-term objective stated?	Yes	No
8. Does baseline information result in identification of deficits in behavior?	Yes	No
C. Structure of the Curriculum		
1. Are specific implementation (presentation) procedures stated?	Yes	No
2. Are the directions for teaching the skills and concepts understandable to you?	Yes	No
3. Are the short-term objectives stated in a hierarchy from simple to complex (sequenced)?	Yes	No
4. Are the short-term objectives dependent or independent of each other (can objectives be extracted from the curriculum and utilized independently or are they prerequisites to each other)?	Yes	No
5. Is the curriculum developed to ensure short learning tasks, frequent review, and frequent testing?	Yes	No
D. Data Collection and Progress Assessment		
1. Are techniques for measurement of client progress specifically stated?	Yes	No
2. Are measurement procedures clear and understandable to you (e.g., are specific behaviors for meeting criteria stated operationally)?	Yes	No

(continued)

Table 13-1. (*continued*)

Evaluation Item	Scoring	
3. Are data sheets for recording and assessing progress provided?	Yes	No
4. Can progress and/or deterioration in clients' behaviors be monitored daily? Weekly? Monthly?	Yes	No
5. Are mastery criteria for each short-term objective specifically stated?	Yes	No
E. Maintenance of Acquired Skills		
1. Does the curriculum provide for periodic monitoring of acquired skills on a *regular* basis (e.g., at least weekly)?	Yes	No
2. Are provisions made for frequent testing (practice) and review of acquired skills?	Yes	No
3. Are specific criteria stated for re-entry into the training program?	Yes	No
4. Does the curriculum specify what training should follow the acquisition of a skill?	Yes	No
5. Are criteria for termination of the maintenance portion of the curriculum specified?	Yes	No
F. Validation of the Curriculum		
1. Was the curriculum field tested?	Yes	No
2. Are the characteristics of the population sample on which the curriculum was field tested identified (e.g., age, sex, disabilities, capabilities)?	Yes	No
3. Are the characteristics of the training setting in which the curriculum was field tested identified (e.g., resource room, special education class, activity center, institution)?	Yes	No
4. Do your clients' characteristics resemble the characteristics of the population sample on which the curriculum was field tested?	Yes	No
G. Practical Considerations		
1. Is the purchase of the curriculum package within your budgetary limitations?	Yes	No
2. Are all necessary materials included or do you have to purchase additional materials?	Yes	No
3. Are the materials that are provided durable?	Yes	No
4. Are the consumable materials reproducible?	Yes	No
5. Is the teaching mode of the curriculum specified in terms of physical facilities needed?	Yes	No
6. Do you have the physical facilities to accommodate the teaching mode?	Yes	No
7. Is the amount of time (per day or per week) that must be devoted to the curriculum in order for it to be effective specified?	Yes	No

Table 13-1. (*continued*)

Evaluation Item	Scoring	
8. Is the staff/client ratio for effective implementation specified?	Yes	No
9. Are instructor prerequisite skills specified?	Yes	No
10. Do the staff who will be using the curriculum have those skills?	Yes	No
11. Is the preparation time of the instructor (to obtain proficiency) specified?	Yes	No
12. Are the materials designed for independent use by the clients?	Yes	No

1. When is it most beneficial to introduce new learning tasks?
2. How should the class be organized, in terms of size and groupings, to effectively teach particular objectives?
3. When should the instructor change strategies if a client is having difficulty acquiring a skill?
4. When is it most beneficial to provide physical or verbal prompts?

The answers to these types of questions will be dependent upon the particular short-term objectives the client is attempting to learn. This information will aid the teacher in troubleshooting and maintaining smooth progression through the curriculum.

A second area of concern is the curriculum's adaptability. Are the short-term objectives dependent on or independent of each other? For example, is the trainer able to extract a particular short-term objective from its sequential position in the curriculum for independent use in another area of the curriculum? (Can the short-term objective of learning to "sweep" be as readily applied to sweeping the kitchen in a residential program as to cleaning the work station, or does the curriculum teach the skill of sweeping by different methods depending on the particular program?) The obvious question is: Can the skills learned in one portion of the curriculum also be applied in another portion of the curriculum? The answers to these types of questions give the teacher an indication of the curriculum's adaptability. Whether you require an adaptable curriculum will depend on the relative needs of the instructors and clients involved. Another way to ask this question is: Does the trainer need a very structured program that specifies step-by-step advancement through the curriculum? Or does the instructor need particular short-term objectives (and methods to reach those objectives) that can be integrated into existing programs? If portions of the curriculum are dependent on each other, the teacher may not be able to extract portions for independent use in some other area.

A few additional questions regarding program implementation need to be addressed here. Smooth progression through a curriculum is dependent on a number of factors. To what degree does the curriculum provide for short learning tasks, frequent review, and frequent testing? These procedures accomplish at least three goals. First, short learning tasks will increase the probability that the student will progress smoothly from one short-term objective to another. This is accomplished by teaching skills that the learner will master in a relatively short time. If the skill is too complicated and lengthy, the client will be unable to master the skill within this short time frame. This only adds to the frustration and experience of failure the individual faces. Second, frequent review provides additional learning trials for the student in order to maintain newly acquired skills. Third, frequent testing (while providing additional learning trials for the student) will provide the teacher with quantitative information regarding the client's progression through the curriculum. Specifically, does the instructor feel the learner should be progressing at a faster rate? This information provides the teacher with a guide on how and when to adapt a curriculum to accommodate the special needs of the individual. For example, if the client is not attaining a particular short-term objective, perhaps the learning task needs to be task analyzed into smaller steps.

Data Collection and Progress Assessment   The merit of any curriculum should be judged by its ability to facilitate skill acquisition. Therefore, a curriculum should provide specific techniques for assessing clients' progress. These measurement procedures should be clear and understandable to the trainer. A curriculum should also identify the criteria for mastery of specific short-term objectives. For example, does the curriculum provide data sheets for recording and assessing progress? Can progress be monitored from these data sheets on a daily basis? Weekly? Monthly? Can deterioration in skills be monitored as closely? When the curriculum is designed to provide this type of information, staff will be better equipped to react to the temporary setbacks that occur in training.

Maintenance of Acquired Skills   Once the client has acquired a given skill, it is extremely important that the new skill be maintained. The curriculum should specify periodic monitoring of newly acquired skills to ensure that the client maintains the ability to perform the skills. This procedure may involve separate times set aside for maintenance checks (e.g., once a month assessment of newly acquired skills to determine if the client still possesses them). Or, it may provide for maintenance checks on skills within the more advanced portions of the curriculum. For example, an instructor may determine if the learner still possesses the skill of making coffee while he/she is involved in dinner preparation.

Periodic monitoring of newly acquired skills need not be a complicated or time-consuming task for the trainer. An additional data sheet for periodic maintenance checks may facilitate this process. The important point is that the newly acquired skills should be monitored to ensure that the client is still capable of demonstrating them. This process is extremely important when the instructor teaches a skill that may not be utilized directly for a few months. For example, assume that your goal is to teach what to do in case of a fire. However, this is only one of many skills you will be teaching. It may be several months before the student has to exhibit this skill while actually engaging in a fire drill. Fire escape procedures should therefore be periodically monitored to ensure that they remain a part of the client's repertoire. If the learner's skill level deteriorates during these maintenance checks, you may wish to retrain the skill to the specified criteria so that further deterioration does not occur.

Validation of the Curriculum   The validation of recently developed materials has received little attention from commercial curriculum developers. Yet, the validity of a curriculum is extremely important when assessing its utility.

The curriculum should indicate whether or not it has been field tested. If the curriculum has not been field tested, you should be aware that it is therefore only experimental in nature. This does not necessarily mean that the curriculum is of no value. It does mean, however, that you need to take additional care in maintaining comprehensive data to verify (or not verify) the curriculum's usefulness.

If the curriculum has been field tested, additional concerns arise. For example, are the characteristics of the population sample on which the curriculum was field tested identified in terms of age, sex, disabilities, capabilities, etc.? In addition, determine whether or not these characteristics are similar to the characteristics of your clients. The more similar the characteristics of these two groups, the more utility the curriculum probably has for you.

The characteristics of the training setting in which the curriculum was field tested should also be identified (e.g., special education classroom, institution). Again, the more similar these characteristics are to the situation in which the curriculum will be applied, the greater the probability that the curriculum will be of benefit.

The answers to these questions will not guarantee that the curriculum is in fact valid. However, they will give you some assurances about the general utility of the curriculum within your setting.

Practical Considerations   Once a decision has been made to purchase materials, the instructor has to consider the economic realities of his or her agency. Several questions need to be answered:

1. Is the cost of the curriculum within budgetary limitations?
2. Are all necessary materials included with the curriculum, or do additional materials need to be purchased?
3. Are the materials durable?

4. Are the consumable portions of the curriculum reproducible (e.g., data sheets, graphs)?

Answers to these questions will help you, as well as your administrators, determine the cost/benefit ratio of the proposed curriculum.

You will also need to identify the physical facilities required for the successful implementation of the curriculum. Obviously, if the trainer does not have access to physical facilities required by the curriculum, it will be of little value. An additional concern deals with the amount of time required for effective implementation of the curriculum. Examples of questions reflecting this concern are:

1. Does the curriculum specify general time and effort requirements for effective implementation?
2. Are you able to invest the time and effort required?
3. Is the instructor/client ratio for effective implementation of the curriculum specified?

These concerns may or may not be within your control. However, this does not detract from the necessity for addressing such considerations.

Another area of concern is the skills required for effective use of the curriculum. For example, does the curriculum identify instructor prerequisite skills? Many curricula assume minimum trainer skill levels for effective implementation. In addition, does the curriculum provide guidelines for the acquisition of skills the teacher may not currently possess? Does the curriculum specify the preparation time required for the instructor prior to effective implementation of the program? It is hoped that the answers to these questions will provide the trainer with meaningful information concerning the feasibility of incorporating a particular curriculum into the existing program.

Using the Checklist

There is no formula for using this checklist that specifies the criteria for selection of materials. Each agency must establish its own criteria. That is, we don't say so many "no" responses means do not purchase materials, so many "yes" responses means purchase the materials. Instead, it is suggested that any questions that receive negative responses be carefully considered prior to the final decision about using materials. Obviously some questions are more critical than others. For example, the first question—"Do the goals and objectives of the curriculum meet your clients' needs as indicated by their long-term goals and their short-term objectives?"—is extremely important. A "no" response to this question would strongly indicate that the materials in question will not meet your programming needs. On the other hand, a "no" response to the question "Are the materials provided durable?" would not necessarily cause you to eliminate the materials from consideration.

Exercise

13-1. Review the checklist, and select those questions to which you feel you must have positive responses in order to adopt materials.

Answers to Exercise

13-1. The following list is a sample of critical questions.
   a. Do the goals and objectives of the curriculum meet your clients' needs as indicated by their long-term goals and short-term objectives?
   b. Do the staff who will be using the curriculum have the skills?
   c. Does the curriculum specifically state long-term goals?
   d. Does the curriculum specifically state short-term objectives?
   e. Are the short-term objectives task analyzed within the curriculum?
   f. Does the curriculum make provision for assessing the clients' skills across the relevant domains?
   g. Are techniques for measurement of client progress specifically stated?
   h. Can progress and/or deterioration in clients' behaviors be monitored?
   i. Was the curriculum field tested?

ADAPTING INSTRUCTIONAL MATERIALS

Although there are many advantages to using instructional materials in your programming, all materials will not necessarily be appropriate for each learner's needs. It may therefore become necessary to adapt materials to match both the objectives defined in the habilitation program and specific learning characteristics of the client. This can be accomplished by adding to the existing resource, changing parts of it, or eliminating certain aspects of it.

Adding to Instructional Materials

Many times, curriculum materials may not include all the instructional tasks your clients need, or appropriate measurement procedures. In these instances, the trainer must supplement the existing resources in order to achieve maximum effectiveness from the materials. For example, the objectives of the curriculum may be too global, and therefore need to be expanded by developing additional behavioral objectives that relate specifically to client needs (Stowitschek et al., 1980). Instructional objectives may omit steps or take steps that are too large for your clients' levels of functioning. A possible solution would be to complete a more extensive task analysis for that particular skill.

In cases when assessment procedures are not included, and the agency decides that the materials still warrant selection, development of recording sheets for each instructional objective with procedures for their use is indicated. Additionally, assessment devices from other materials can be used. Another common limitation of materials is the absence of practical activities to strengthen the acquired behavior. Again, how often to monitor and the method of monitoring practical activities could be added.

Changing Materials

In some instances the instructional materials may need to be modified in either format or presentation. For example, in a self-instructional package where learners independently use the resource, instructions for the completion of a task are provided in a complex written form. This may need to be changed to single word instructions or to auditory instructions via tape recorder. Another common limitation is the required mode of training that the instructor is to use in working with the client. For example, the materials may provide only verbal directions with the required task. Depending upon the individual client, this may need to be changed to verbal plus physical prompts. Other items that may be changed in curricula are sequence of task analysis, the way in which a prompt is delivered (e.g., visual, auditory), and recording sheets.

Deleting Aspects of the Program

When a part of the program is inappropriate for a particular client, you have the option of discarding it. A detailed task analysis may be given for a dressing skill. If the client knows how to perform some of the steps, it would be unnecessary to go through them. For example, suppose you have a task analysis for putting on pants, which includes learning how to zip. The client may know how to zip his pants, but cannot put them on. In this instance, the trainer does not have to teach the skill of zipping but simply makes sure it is presented in the appropriate sequence. Frequently tasks are eliminated from a curriculum because the particular skill is either not appropriate for the client *or* not within the agency's realm to deliver. For example, in a comprehensive curriculum on vocational training skills, there exists a section on table saw operation. Obviously, if your agency did not possess this equipment, this section of the curriculum could be deleted.

The most important thing to remember in using instructional resources is to individualize the materials to fit client needs. This is accomplished by: 1) identifying the goals and objectives of a habilitation program, 2) systematically reviewing existing resources, 3) selecting materials to use, 4) adapting these materials according to client's needs, and 5) evaluating the effectiveness of the instructional package in promoting client growth (Stowitschek et al., 1980).

DESIGNING INSTRUCTIONAL MATERIALS

Designing instructional materials is extremely difficult, and the authors suggest that it should be considered only when no other resources are available. Creating new materials for use in habilitation programming must begin with an analysis of needs of particular clients and identification of the goals and objectives of the program plans. It is suggested that individuals who are interested in developing their own materials contact a professional in the area of curriculum design for assistance.

SUGGESTED ACTIVITIES

Take a curriculum that your facility is currently using and evaluate it using the checklist. If the curriculum did not meet acceptable standards, decide how you would adapt it.

ADDITIONAL RESOURCES

Brown, V. A basic Q sheet for analyzing and comparing curriculum materials and proposals. *Journal of Learning Disabilities,* 1975, *8*(7), 409–416.

Henderson, H., & Rouig, T. Evaluating, selecting and adapting instructional materials: A critical teacher competency. *NSPI Journal,* July 1977, 18–23.

Kaufman, R. A. *Educational system planning.* Englewood Cliffs, N.J.: Prentice-Hall, 1972.

Meyen, S. L. *Developing instructional units: Applications for the exceptional child.* Dubuque, Iowa: Brown, 1976.

REFERENCES

Czajkowski, L., Zawitkowski, A., & Pearce, L. *Directions in adapted physical education.* Vermillion, S.D.: Center for the Developmentally Disabled, University of South Dakota, 1980.

Stowitschek, J., Gable, R., & Hendrickson, J. *Instructional materials for exceptional children: Selection, management and adaptation.* Germantown, Md.: Aspen Publications, 1980.

Unit VI

The Proactive Organization
Support for Going

Chapter 14

Administrative Skills and Strategies

OBJECTIVES

To be able to:
1. Describe the five main managerial styles defined by Blake and Mouton.
2. Compare your own managerial behavior to styles described in the managerial grid.
3. List the advantages and disadvantages of each of the five managerial styles.
4. Describe how feelings and perceptions affect communication.
5. List the six steps involved in decision making.
6. Construct a program to change one aspect of your own behavior.

The next three chapters take a slightly different focus from what you have read so far. There are several major components to providing effective habilitative services, including the staff, the client, and the agency. These next chapters address the management of the agency and the staff of the agency in which programming occurs. Nothing is more critical to providing successful programming for clients than how staff relate to each other, their superiors, and their subordinates.

The expansion in the number and range of community-based programs in the last 10 years is nothing short of phenomenal. Bruininks, Hauber, and Kudla (1979) noted an increase of 3,816 reporting community residential programs between 1972 and 1977. This increase in the number of programs has been accompanied by a similar increase in the number of staff, primarily at the direct care level. A recent survey estimates that there are 80,000 "paraprofessionals" in educational programs alone (Humm, 1980). This growth in programs and staff has resulted in the need for many persons to assume the role of manager or supervisor for a program.

Pfriem (1980) found that the majority of direct care staff enter programs with little or no prior experience or appropriate education for the requirements of the job. This is largely true for program managers and supervisors in most community-based programs. A survey of developmental disability managers completed by Gettings (personal communication, November 1980) found that only 5.2% of the respondents had a degree in business; however, most had advanced degrees (master's or doctorate) in a clinical area (e.g., psychology, speech pathology). This situation is in part a result of the newness of community-based programs and in part because human services agencies have long selected or promoted persons for reasons having nothing to do with managerial skill. Promotion typically occurs because of recognized skill at a lower level in the hierarchy (e.g., a good nurse is promoted to nurse supervisor) or longevity within the field or organization. The central themes of this unit are that program managers are made, not born or promoted, and that management skills can be identified, operationalized, and put into practice with measurable results. The purpose of this chapter is to acquaint you with the problems that occur when bosses collide with the bossed.

One commonly accepted definition of management is "the process of getting work done through others" (Duncan, 1973). This implies that management is concerned with a product (getting work done) and with people (others), and that management is in a position to direct the performance of others. Blake and Mouton (1964) have identified three organization universals:

1. Purpose—what product you produce.
2. People—who produce and constitute an organization.
3. Hierarchy—simply put, some people are bosses and some people are bossed. The achievement of organizational purpose results in hierarchy.

MANAGERIAL STYLES

Managerial behavior can be viewed as an interaction among these three organizational universals. Thus, a manager may vary in his or her concern for production, concern for people, and how he or she perceives the hierarchial nature of an organization.

The Managerial Grid® (Blake & Mouton, 1964, 1978) shows the possible interactions between concern for people and concern for production (Figure 14-1). Placement on the Grid carries implications for a manager's hierarchical behavior as well. Each "concern" is represented by a 9-point scale, with 1 being low concern and 9 maximum concern. A total of 81 combinations of managerial behavior is possible on the Grid; the five represented show the most distinct sets of assumptions regarding how bosses manage people. Blake

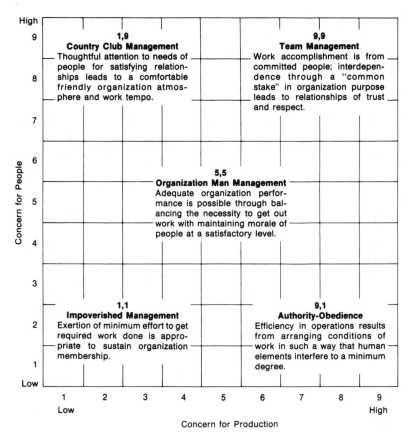

Figure 14-1. The Managerial Grid. (Reprinted by permission from: Blake, R., & Mouton, J. *The Managerial Grid*. Houston: Gulf Publishing Co., 1978.)

and Mouton (1978) suggest that for any person there is a dominant style and backup styles of management. Thus, an individual is rarely rigidly fixed in any one management style. The particular style that is evident at any time is a function of several variables:

1. *Organization*—many organizational factors, such as rigidity of procedures, can affect a manager's behavior.
2. *Situation*—managerial behavior in certain situations, such as a high-stress crisis, may be different than in routine transactions.
3. *Values*—managerial behavior may be based on a manager's belief concerning the "right" way to treat people.
4. *Personality*—long-standing characteristics may predispose a manager to prefer a certain style.

5. *Chance*—a manager may choose a certain style as a result of unfamiliarity with other styles.

It is important to note that managerial styles are not fixed but are subject to influence from a variety of sources.

The 9,1 Managerial Style

The 9,1 manager (see Figure 14-1) has a high concern for production and a low concern for people. In an extreme case, the 9,1 manager is hard driving and completely involved in one organizational universal: production. The managerial style is rather autocratic, because the 9,1 manager utilizes his or her position of superiority within the organizational hierarchy to make most, if not all, decisions. The relationship to subordinates is characterized by dominance and obedience. Subordinates need to be dominated and obedient because the 9,1 manager believes that people do not like or want to work. The 9,1 manager believes that conflict occurs because of "soft" leadership. Therefore, directives are stern, communication is reduced to the bare essentials (and generally in written terms), and conflict within the organization is suppressed. That in no way suggests that conflict is nonexistent. Rather, it is displaced by workers and oftentimes rearises indirectly. This is known as antiorganizational creativity, where staff find indirect methods to fight the system.

Blake and Mouton (1964) suggest that one consequence of 9,1 management is unionization. Another consequence is increased government intervention as management is unable to cope with organizational problems. Furthermore, workers are less productive because management fails to develop, tap, and maintain a valuable resource.

The 1,9 Managerial Style

Interestingly enough, the 1,9 manager shares some characteristics with the 9,1 manager. While high on concern for people, and low on concern for production, the 1,9 manager is similar in the sense that management will provide the structure and motivation for workers, and works to minimize conflict. What differs is the 1,9 manager's *method* of approaching these assumptions. The 1,9 manager wants to be accepted by subordinates. Therefore, by promoting camaraderie, smoothing over criticism, and promoting company spirit, he or she can avoid personal rejection. This style of management has also been referred to as the "country club style."

Supervisor-subordinate relationships are paternal in nature (one big happy family), and characterized by an avoidance of conflict ("if you can't say anything nice. . . ."). The creation of high morale is thought to be the key to a good organization because people do not like to work. Thus, the 1,9 manager believes morale is increased via favors (taking time off to watch special events on TV), pleasant working conditions (coffee and doughnuts), and high supervisor visibility (frequent "chats").

The 1,9 approach, which does not allow for organizational conflict, can lead to happy interpersonal relationships. However, production typically suffers through a lack of clear expectations and performance feedback.

The 1,1 Managerial Style

Low concern for both people and production characterize the 1,1 manager. It seems to be a contradiction in terms to conceive of an individual with low concerns in both areas surviving with an organization. Actually, such survival is considered an art form (James Boren has written an excellent book describing the 1,1 style, entitled *When in Doubt, Mumble*).

The 1,1 is more of a nonperson within the organization. The person comes to work and appears busy, but is rarely seen as an active, visible boss. Minimum control is exercised over both people and production and there is virtually no decision-making. Blake and Mouton (1964) provide the following account of a 1,1 manager's interactions with subordinates:

> The supervisor had just returned from a weekly staff meeting, where changes in procedures, policies and the like are discussed so that each subordinate can initiate appropriate changes within his own area of responsibility. The supervisor, as was his usual custom, called his five subordinates to his office. When all were seated, he read mechanically a copy of a memorandum and notes he had taken as it had been presented earlier and had been discussed. He checked off each topic as he read it, careful that none could say later that he had not "communicated." When he had completed this recitation, he filed the memo and his dated notes in his desk drawer.
> Without looking up, he said, "I'm going to the record shop. Who has the (company car) key?" The keys were located. As he turned to leave, one subordinate ventured a question concerning how and when a particular change was to be effected.
> "They didn't say," was the supervisor's reply.
> Another raised a question about fifteen large boxes of materials in the hallway.
> "They just said to order them. They didn't say what to do with them when they got here. Let them set. Somebody will come get them when they start looking for the stuff." With that, he left. (p. 87)

The 1,1 manager seeks to isolate himself or herself from contact with both superiors and subordinates, although he or she generally follows company policy to the letter (staff meetings once a week whether we need them or not). There is no organizational creativity, because all efforts are directed at personal survival. Conflict is avoided whenever possible.

In business, which must be accountable for productivity, few 1,1 styles exist for any long period. However, in government programs with numerous built-in protections against firing, or in loosely monitored programs with poorly specified expectancies, 1,1 managers can and do flourish. The 1,1 managerial style is unique in that, rather than being a style an individual enters an organization with, the 1,1 style seems to be a response to personal defeat that an individual develops over time.

The 5,5 Managerial Style

The basic assumption of the 5,5 manager is to not idealistically seek to maximize people or production, but to compromise. The 5,5 manager believes himself or herself to be seeking the best of both worlds. While reserving the responsibility for planning, directing, and controlling the organization, the 5,5 manager also seeks to be understood by and receive input from subordinates. The 5,5 manager acts as a "fixer" if problems arise. Thus, the 5,5 performs a delicate balancing act between conflicting interests in his or her effort to maintain a smoothly running organization.

The 5,5 manager prefers a one-to-one style of superior-subordinate interactions, and is likely to be perceived by subordinates as a "regular guy." When a particular task arises, committees or study groups that make recommendations to the manager are generally utilized. In this fashion, the 5,5 manager allows a form of participatory management without giving up authority.

Conflict is not particularly suppressed nor encouraged. However, it is the 5,5 manager who wants to be the solver of conflict. Because he or she recognizes people as important, the 5,5 manager uses a splitting-the-difference approach to conflict resolution. Thus, if one employee prefers hot, and another prefers cold, the 5,5 manager will seek resolution by providing both employees with lukewarm or 3½ days each of hot and cold. One problem here is that now neither staff member is satisfied, and the manager has two disgruntled employees.

The 5,5 manager is perhaps the one most commonly found in American business today (Whyte, 1955; Blake & Mouton, 1964). Although this is not a particularly evil approach, the controlling aspects and methods of conflict resolution do have the effect of lowering productivity and reducing creativity.

The 9,9 Managerial Style

The basis of the 9,9 approach to management is to view people and organizations as not inherently in conflict. Rather, conflicts arise through the management of people to achieve organizational needs.

The heart of the 9,9 manager's approach includes clear delineation and delegation of responsibility and authority within the organization, a utilization of the team approach, and an encouragement of open conflict resolution. The 9,9 manager views his or her job as facilitating communication and decision-making within the organization. This facilitation is viewed as distinctly different from actually *making* the decisions or being the origin of communication.

Napier and Gershenfeld (1973) describe three assumptions that are characteristic of managers who utilize the 9,9 style:

1. If the actual sources of tension are not uncovered and dealt with, it is highly likely that they will be diffused into other areas.
2. Unless individuals feel free to express themselves within the problem-solving situation, they will respond with characteristic defensiveness.
3. Often, the issues causing conflict are personal and emotional, while discussion remains technical. Discussion must address the issues.

Additionally, the 9,9 manager's reliance on the team approach is founded on the assumption that informed groups usually make better decisions than individuals, and that those involved in making the decision usually will have a higher stake in implementation (Johnson & Johnson, 1975). The long-term effects of 9,9 management on an organization are increased profitability, improved interpersonal relationships, strengthened teams, and increased individual creativity. Clearly, the 9,9 approach results in a productive committed work force.

For a more complete explanation of the grid approach to managerial behavior see Blake and Mouton (1964, 1978).

COMMUNICATION

As we have seen, the 9,9 manager serves as a facilitator in production and decision-making. This facilitator role means that the ability to effectively communicate is very important to any manager. Blake and Mouton (1968) surveyed managers in three countries and found that communication difficulties were perceived as the key barriers to effective organizational functioning by 63% of managers in Great Britain, 74% in the United States, and 85% in Japan. In fact, it is realistic to state that good management and good communication are synonymous. Indeed, as a supervisor moves up the management hierarchy, increasing amounts of time are spent in communication. This is one problem facing the technical expert who is thrust into management positions: the skills necessary to perform the new job are different and largely unrelated to the old. In fact, a study by Maier, Hoffman, and Read (1963) indicates that previously holding a subordinate's job does not necessarily make the superior better at communicating with the subordinate.

Generally speaking, we take communication for granted. This is unfortunate because it is an extremely complex process, which can be derailed at any one of a number of points. We communicate (manage) for results (production), and poor communication can be destructive to organizational effectiveness.

The communication process can be represented as shown in Figure 14-2. All messages have a source (S), and the thoughts of the sender have to be

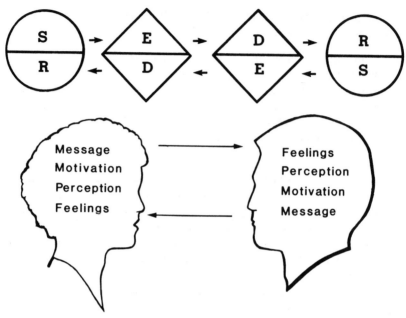

Figure 14-2. The communication process. S, source of message; E, encoding of sender's thoughts; D, decoding of sender's thoughts; R, receiver.

encoded (E) in a transmittable form (communication via verbal, nonverbal, written, or other like means). The message is then decoded (D) by the receiver (R), and particular "meanings" are attached to the message. It is in the decoding and encoding of messages that the process breaks down, because the meaning of a given message is partially based on the feelings and perceptions of the sender and receiver.

To increase the effectiveness of communication, a manager must first be aware of some of the barriers that interfere with the process:

1. Differences in education, experience, and cultural background are inherent in the multidisciplinary, programmatically variable services for the developmentally disabled. These differences can create tremendous barriers to effective communication.

2. Lack of information can cause difficulties in achieving expected results. For example, new program regulations may demand a level of expertise not currently present in staff.

3. The words themselves can lead to distortion of messages. Developmental disabilities is full of jargon (DD, SSDI, ACMRDD, IPP, RSA) that, for the uninitiated, is impossible to understand.

4. Personal bias, which we accept as the "norm" and thus do not perceive as a barrier to communication, can interfere with effective sending and receiving.

5. Poor listening habits (e.g., daydreaming, tuning out before hearing the full message) lead to a lack of understanding. [For an excellent discussion of listening skills, see Deunk (1967).]

In addition to awareness, effective communication involves actively overcoming these barriers by evaluating our own strengths and weaknesses as managers, as well as those of subordinates. First, decide precisely what you *want* to *occur* before you send a message. Specifying a particular outcome will help determine how (method), what (message), and when (timing) to communicate, and to whom. Next, encourage feedback from receivers. Do not assume a message is received just because it was sent. We can all think of examples in our own behavior when the first line of a memo was read and then discarded. Finally, work at being a good listener yourself. Concentrate, make eye contact, and give feedback. Modeling good communication skills can increase the effectiveness of others within the organization.

DECISION-MAKING

Good decision-making ability is one of the most important skills a manager can possess. Total organizational effectiveness, including planning, staffing patterns, programs, expansion, and productivity, is directly related to the effectiveness of the decisions made by the organization. Moreover, the quality of care that clients receive appears to be related to staff involvement in the decision-making process (King, Raynes, & Tizard, 1971; Raynes, Pratt, & Roses, 1977).

Griffiths (1959) has outlined steps necessary to effective decision-making. Although following these steps (see Figure 14-3) does not guarantee that all decisions made will prove to be "good," it does increase the probability that decisions will follow from input, adequate examination of possible solutions, and accounting for possible outcomes. Thus, decision-making becomes planned and proactive, and stops resembling the aimless wandering of a tumbleweed blown by any prevailing wind.

Step 1—Perceive and Operationalize the Problem   As repeatedly stated, unless we know where we are, the probability of goal achievement is reduced. Although it is recognized that not all people similarly perceive a given problem, effective managers are better able to sort through and pinpoint exactly where the problem lies.

Exercise

14-1. The residential program recently consulted a behavior management expert to solve a problem. It seems that there was a high recidivism rate for clients promoted to semi-independent living situations from supervised settings. The program requested in-service training for the supervised living staff to help them better prepare clients for promotion. During a pre-training assessment, the consultant discovered that there were no consis-

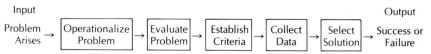

Figure 14-3. The steps to effective decision-making. (Adapted from Griffiths, D. E. *Administrative theory*. New York: Appleton-Century-Crofts, 1959.)

tent exit criteria from supervised living and no entrance criteria for semi-independent living, little communication among staff, and no formal procedures for generalizing training done in supervised to semi-independent living. How would you now perceive the problem?

Step 2—Evaluate the Problem   Ask the following questions: What does the problem mean to me? What does the problem mean to the organization? What does it mean to those affected by it? What do I want to do about it? What do we want to do about it?

Exercise

14-2.   Now that we have decided that the real problem(s) in our residential program described above is that there are no exit or entrance criteria, poor staff communication, and no formal generalization procedures, apply the questions in Step 2. Some of your answers ought to reflect your leadership style (lack of clear direction) and the morale of your staff (morale is probably low if there is a high recidivism rate). What do you want to do about it? If you're following the 9/9 style, your immediate answer ought to be involve the staff.

Step 3—Establish Criteria for Judgment   This is a critical step in decision-making, because values of the individual manager and the organization come heavily into play. In effect, the manager must determine his or her goal, or answer to the question "How will I know if the decision is the right one?"

Exercise

14-3.   What goals will you now set? You've correctly perceived and evaluated the problems in your residential program. Are you really committed to client training? A lower recidivism rate might be one goal.

Step 4—Collect Data   Any decision must be based on collection of all available data. Screen the relevant from the irrelevant, and apply "weights" to each piece of data—some information might be more important than others.

Exercise

14-4.   In the initial request for training, the residential program had accurately identified one big problem (recidivism rate) but had hastily decided on a solution before collecting the relevant data. How would you go about collecting such data? The consultant in this case utilized two important methods. First, she talked extensively to staff of both programs, and, second, she had knowledge of successful programs. She was able to compare this program with successful programs and thereby identify differences. You are now ready to move to solve the problem in Step 5.

Step 5—Select the Preferred Solution   This step is actually made up of three smaller substeps. In order to select the preferred solution, a manager should:

1. Formulate several solutions.
2. Anticipate the advantages and disadvantages of each prospective "solution."
3. Select the solution most likely to succeed.

Step 6—Implement the Solution   When implementing the solution, a manager must also be prepared to modify the solution in the face of feedback about the solution's effectiveness or lack thereof.

SELF-CONTROL—MANAGING THE MANAGER

As we have seen in previous chapters, environmental contingencies and environmental manipulations produce well-documented effects on behavior. These parameters are more immediately observable, more accessible to manipulation, easier to replicate, and as a result more open to direct test than any internal controls that a person may utilize in directing behavior (Ziarnik, 1977). The proactive administrator must seek to manage his or her own behavior, and application of the principles of learning discussed in the previous chapters can help manage time, change interpersonal behaviors with employees and supervisors, and make job behaviors increasingly productive.

Self-control procedures have been used to modify a wide variety of behaviors, such as excessive cigarette smoking (McFall, 1970; Berecz, 1972), repeated and troublesome thoughts (Johnson, 1971), and weight loss (Hall, 1972), and have even been applied to the excessive behaviors of children (Bolstad & Johnson, 1971).

The term "self-control" refers to any instance of self-imposed behavior change. Kanfer and Phillips (1970) detailed several factors that seem to be important in effective self-control:

1. *Self-monitoring.*   Just as with a client, you have to know where you are before you begin a program. Self-monitoring is simply counting your own behavior. Counting can be accomplished via the same methods utilized for clients (see Chapter 6), including wrist counters and paper and pencil. But, beware: people tend to be inaccurate when self-monitoring.
2. *Manipulation of the environment.*   Examine *when* and *where* you do or don't do a particular behavior. As with a client, you are identifying environmental cues, or those that increase the likelihood of behaving in a

certain way. Imagine that you wished to change the time frame in which you answered letters. First, you might want to look at where you file them to be answered and how long it takes to answer them. Changing might involve a special "letter-answering hour."

3. *Label the behavior.* This involves accurate identification of what you wish to change and operationalization of the behavior.

4. *Provide self-reinforcement.* First, you need to know what you enjoy. Next, begin to engage in these activities contingent upon doing things not quite as pleasurable.

SUGGESTED ACTIVITIES

1. Suppose your staff indicated that they wanted you to increase your rate of positive reinforcement for their activities. Construct a self-control program to change this behavior.

2. List the top ten activities you like to do. Then count how many times you do these over a week. Low frequency? Maybe you need to take more control of your reinforcers.

3. Define your product. Operationalize your agency's product in terms you would expect from a client's IPP.

4. Complete the time management checklist on pages 274–276. This time control checklist was developed by Drs. Bill Garove and Tom Fenekes. If you have a low score, you need to read these books: Lakein, A., *How to get control of your time and your life,* New York: New American Library, Inc., 1974; and MacKenzie, R. A., *The time trap,* New York: Amacom Publishers, 1972.

ADDITIONAL RESOURCES

Blake, R., & Mouton, J. *The managerial Grid.* Houston: Gulf Publishing Co., 1964.
   This is the first of a series of grid books. Clearly written, it is an excellent place for a manager to begin.

Blake, R., & Mouton, J. *The new managerial Grid.* Houston: Gulf Publishing Co., 1978.
   In this expanded and revised version, Blake and Mouton expand on applications of the Grid and take a firmer position regarding the necessity of the 9,9 approach.

AUDIOVISUAL MATERIALS

Communication: The non-verbal agenda. Delmar, Calif.: CRM Productions, McGraw-Hill Films, 1974. (16 mm)
   An excellent film! Everytime we see this, we notice something new. One of the best communication films around.

What do you mean, what do I mean? Santa Monica, Calif.: Salenger Educational Media, 1974. (16 mm)
   An excellent film with vignettes and structured discussion around how communication goes wrong.

REFERENCES

Berecz, J. Modification of smoking behavior through self-administered punishment of imagined behavior: A new approach to aversive therapy. *Journal of Consulting and Clinical Psychology,* 1972, *38,* 244–250.

Blake, R. R., & Mouton, J. S. *The managerial grid.* Houston: Gulf Publishing Co., 1964.

Blake, R. R., & Mouton, J. S. *Grid organizational development.* Houston: Gulf Publishing Co., 1968.

Blake, R. R., & Mouton, J. S. *The new managerial grid.* Houston: Gulf Publishing Co., 1978.

Bolstad, O., & Johnson, S. M. Self-regulation in the modification of disruptive behavior. *Journal of Applied Behavior Analysis,* 1971, *4*(3), 191–199.

Bruininks, R. H., Hauber, R. A., & Kudla, M. J. *National survey of community residential facilities: A profile of facilities and residents in 1977* (project report No. 5). Minneapolis: University of Minnesota Developmental Disabilities Project on Residential Services and Community Adjustment, December 1979.

Deunk, H. H. Active listening: A forgotten key to effective communication. *Hospital Administration,* Spring, 1967.

Duncan, C. *Managing for results.* Atlanta: U.S. Department of Health, and Welfare, Public Health Service, Center for Disease Control, 1973.

Griffiths, D. E. *Administrative theory.* New York: Appleton-Century-Crofts, 1959.

Hall, S. M. Self-control and therapist control in the behavioral treatment of overweight women. *Behavior Research and Therapy,* 1972, *10,* 59–68.

Humm, A. *New directions newsletter.* New Careers Training Laboratory, 1980, *2*(1).

Johnson, D. W., & Johnson, F. P. *Joining together: Group theory and skills.* Englewood Cliffs, N.J.: Prentice-Hall, 1975.

Johnson, W. G. Some applications of Hommes' coverant control therapy: Two case reports. *Behavior Therapy,* 1971, *2,* 240–248.

Kanfer, F. H., & Phillips, J. S. *Learning foundations of behavior therapy.* New York: John Wiley & Sons, 1970.

King, R. D., Raynes, N. V., & Tizard, J. *Patterns of residential care: Sociological studies in institutions for handicapped citizens.* London: Routledge & Kegan Paul, 1971.

McFall, R. M. The affects of self-monitoring on normal smoking behavior. *Journal of Consulting and Clinical Psychology,* 1970, *35,* 135–146.

Maier, N. R. F., Hoffman, R. L., & Read, W. H. Superior-subordinate communication: The relative effectiveness of managers who held their subordinates' positions. *Personnel Psychology,* 1963, *16,* 1–11.

Napier, R., & Gershenfeld, M. K. *Groups: Theory and experience.* Boston: Houghton Mifflin Co., 1973.

Pfriem, D. *Tinker to Evers but no Chance: Staff training as a cooperative effort.* Presented at the American Association on Mental Deficiency, San Francisco, 1980.

Raynes, N. V., Pratt, M. W., & Roses, S. Aides' involvement in decision-making and the quality of care in institutional settings. *American Journal of Mental Deficiency,* 1977, *81,* 570–577.

Whyte, W. F. *Money and motivation.* New York: Harper, 1955.

Ziarnik, J. P. The relative efficacy of in-vivo self monitoring and video tape feedback in altering rates of question-asking in group therapists. *Dissertation Abstracts International,* 1977, *37*(11-B), 6359.

Time Control Checklist for Busy Developmental Disabilities Managers[a]

The following exercise should help you gain insight into the degree of control you have on your job and the related results. A subtle way of placing your job in perspective is by assessing it conscientiously with the use of time as a resource.

The process of running a time check can be a profitable technique. Use the checklist below. Check the column at the right that best describes your behavior in regard to each given statement.

Following completion of the checklist, ask your secretary or a colleague to evaluate you, using this same checklist.

	Always	Sometimes	Never
1. Do you keep in mind the cost of one hour of your time?	——	——	——
2. Do you weigh the time requirements of a task prior to assigning it to others or undertaking it yourself?	——	——	——
3. Do you jot down ideas and important facts when they come to mind, rather than relying on memory?	——	——	——
4. Does paperwork take up a minimum portion of your work day?	——	——	——
5. Do you use "stock paragraphs" in your letters to cover "stock" situations?	——	——	——
6. Do you give explicit instructions when assigning tasks?	——	——	——
7. Do you have your secretary maintain a monthly-yearly calendar of events involving you?	——	——	——
8. Do you brief your secretary weekly on your schedule of events?	——	——	——
9. Do you use periodic meetings or individual conferences with subordinates for setting objectives and goals and reviewing their performances?	——	——	——
10. Do you handwrite a note of appreciation or recognition periodically to your subordinates for an outstanding achievement?	——	——	——
11. Do you approach major decisions with an organized problem-solving strategy? (Identifying the problem clearly, listing alternative solutions and analyzing each solution in terms of its consequences)	——	——	——
12. Are you aware of when you are procrastinating?	——	——	——
13. Do you limit time spent with each visitor? (Expected or unexpected)	——	——	——
14. Do you anticipate possible problems and devise strategies to prevent them?	——	——	——
15. Do you exercise close control over your telephone conversations?	——	——	——
16. Do you make the best use of others' time at meetings, conferences, etc.?	——	——	——

(continued)

Time Control Checklist *(continued)*

REMEMBER, HAVE YOUR SECRETARY OR A COLLEAGUE EVALUATE YOU,
USING THE SAME CHECKLIST.

Now that you have completed the time control checklist follow the directions
given below.
1. Count the number of checks in the *Always* column and multiply by 5.
2. Count the number of checks placed under the *Sometimes* column and multiply by 3.
3. Total the results of 1 and 2 above and compute your score.
   Enter your score here _____
4. Compare your score with the scale given below:
   61–80   You control your job rather than your job controlling you
   41–60   You have your responsibilities in fair perspective
    0–40   Your job controls you
5. If you would desire to improve your score, the following action is recommended:
   A. Analyze your responses.
   B. Identify those you checked in the *Sometimes* or *Never* columns that:
      1. Seem to make sense to you
      2. Seem like behaviors you would want to change to the "Always"
         column
   C. Prioritize those you have identified in B above according to their *practi-
      cality* and *compatibility* to your job conditions.
   D. Starting with the most practical and compatible one, develop an action
      plan by listing in sequence the steps you will need to take to convert the
      Sometimes/Never response to an Always response. Also note the time
      line you would recommend for yourself. (Below is the format. You may
      want to give yourself more room by using regular blank table paper.)

ACTION PLAN	TIME LINE

   E. Be certain that you develop a means of evaluating your progress on the
      results of your action delineated above.
   F. List who might help you achieve the results and/or the evaluation.
   G. What *obstacles* might you anticipate?
   H. What alternatives can you list to minimize barriers to your progress?
   I. After you have accomplished a regular pattern of behavior with a parti-
      cular time management technique, repeat steps D –I with the remaining
      behaviors you feel you want to improve.

(continued)

Time Control Checklist   (continued)

EXAMPLE:
#8   To develop a procedure for briefing my secretary on my weekly schedule of events.

ACTION PLAN	TIME LINE
1. Meet with secretary and discuss my desire to establish a system of keeping her informed of my weekly activities.	Within 48 hours
2. Discuss with her the rationale why and ask her for suggestions for implementing the plan. Agree on means of evaluation and time line for implementation/evaluate/ confirm.	
3. Implement immediately.	Within 72 hours
4. Evaluate self-behavior/results.	End of full month
5. Request secretary to evaluate results of the implemented behavior and share the same at the predetermined conference.	End of full month

[a] Reprinted by permission from Bill Garove and Tom Fernekes, Management Training Program, School of Community and Allied Health Sciences, University of Alabama, Birmingham. Adapted from: Lagana, J. F. *Time of your life program: Effective time management guidebook.* Pittsburgh, Pa.: Author, 1978.

Chapter 15

Organizational Development and Personnel Management

OBJECTIVES

To be able to:
1. List the eight assumptions underlying organizational development.
2. Write performance objectives.
3. Explain the process involved in developing shared goals between staff and the organization.
4. Distinguish between Herzberg's and Maslow's theories of motivation.
5. Construct a Table of Organization that reflects your organization's functioning.
6. List three reasons for giving performance feedback.
7. List the five steps involved in planned organizational change.

The purpose of the previous chapter was to familiarize managers with a variety of management skills and personal orientations associated with effective organizational functioning. This chapter is designed to present managers with information about organizational development. Also, this chapter can help line staff become more aware of the complex issues involved in a holistic approach to client habilitation. In a general sense, the goal of organizational development is to create a system of people who are able to change as the organization responds to new environmental demands (French, 1969). More specifically, organizational development involves:

1. Long-range planned change based upon a shared perception of need (by the members of the organization).
2. Viewing the entire organization as a system.

3. Creating new awareness about alternative methods of perceiving the organization's ongoing activities.

Many of the techniques, methods, and philosophical premises involved in organizational development (i.e., reinforcement, clear goal setting, data-based decisions, proactive behavior) are not particularly distinct from those outlined in previous chapters in this book. However, if the procedures described in this book are to be effectively implemented for clients, the organizational climate must encourage such behaviors. This book has been concerned with effective habilitative programming for clients. But think about a community-based program for the developmentally disabled for a moment. What comes to mind? A production-oriented business, a sheltered environment, an activities center, a top-notch habilitative program? The image you create for your organization will have a direct relationship to the kind of organization you get and kind of behavior staff exhibit. Thus, there is a tremendous reciprocity between organizations and people. For example, a program viewed as primarily a sheltered workshop or a production-oriented business will likely emphasize production, marketing, and contract procurement. These activities, which are congruent with the organization's needs, will be encouraged in staff. On the other hand, staff of these programs will not be encouraged to place clients outside the agency, or to spend a great deal of individual time with clients. It is a source of much confusion when an organization gives mixed messages to staff.

There are several assumptions underlying the concept of organizational development (Bennis, 1969):

1. The way in which people approach their jobs is more a function of how they are treated by the organization than of any intrinsic personality characteristics they may possess. Therefore, to change work habits, change the organization or change how the organization treats staff.
2. Organizations in which the needs of people and the needs of the organization are similar are most productive.
3. People are motivated by challenging work. They are not motivated by the avoidance of work.
4. Organizations are built on groups of people, not simply individuals.
5. The free expression of ideas is an important aspect of employees becoming committed to a particular task.
6. Groups that can openly provide feedback to group members relative to work tasks are more productive.
7. Commitment, not simply agreement, to do a task is necessary to most fully utilize an organization's resources.
8. Through planned change, data-based objectives, and clear expectations, organizational development seeks to increase the number of choices or options available to an organization.

Let's examine organizational development through a more detailed analysis of these assumptions.

WORK HABITS AND THE ORGANIZATION

Hamerlynck (1980) has suggested that, by and large, the interaction between people and governing organizations primarily involves aversive control and countercontrol. He cites as an example state personnel systems in which it is nearly impossible to make reward (or lack of it) contingent upon job performance. In fact, most personnel policy procedures seem to be designed to have as little to do with job performance as possible. One method an administrator can utilize to more clearly communicate job expectation (and thus, more clearly utilize rewards *contingent* upon good performance) is performance objectives.

Performance Objectives

Statements of goals and objectives for staff are the first step in performance evaluation. Several studies (Burke & Wilcox, 1969; Miner, 1969) indicate that both superiors and subordinates are negatively inclined toward evaluation. That is, supervisors dislike doing it, and staff dislike receiving it. This is in part due to the fact that many performance evaluations are based on vague, unoperationalized concepts: is responsible, dresses neatly, good ethical conduct, and so forth. Couple vague criteria with the fact that managers and workers differ in the criteria that they use in making judgments about people (Triandis, 1959, 1960), and the result is bound to be disastrous. Greene (1972) found that, the more accurately a subordinate complies with a superior's expectation, the higher the subordinate's job satisfaction. Boyd and Jensen (1972) suggest that first-line supervisors and their superiors have difficulty agreeing on the supervisor's authority. The best way to clear up these problems is with a clear, objective, negotiated set of performance objectives for all staff. We suggest the following format[1]:

Time %	Objective	Authority	Date Due	Actual Date

[1]Reprinted by permission from Bill Garove and Tom Fernekes, Management Training Program, School of Community and Allied Health Sciences, University of Alabama, Birmingham.

Time % refers to the actual percentage of time the staff member is expected to devote to the objective. The total of *all* objectives must be 100%.

Objectives are *clear, operationalized* statements regarding job tasks. Refer to previous chapters if you need refreshers about operationalized language.

Authority means who must complete the task. In order to complete a task, staff must not only have responsibility, but authority as well. A good manager delegates authority. Mark A for complete authority; mark B for authority required. What this delineates is whether staff may act independently in pursuit of the objective or whether they have to receive approval from someone.

Date Due is the date the objective is expected to be completed. *Actual Date* refers to when the objective was achieved. Discrepancies can be a basis for discussion between managers and staff.

Sample performance objectives might look like this:

Name: Paula Jones   *Title:* Case Manager   *Date:* September 1980

Time %	Objective	Authority	Date Due	Actual Date
25	To staff and develop IPPs for 30 clients.	A	1–1–81	
35	To monitor, on at least a weekly basis, the progress of each of 30 clients.	A	Continuous	
40	To work with the in-service coordinator to present a minimum of 14 training programs for staff.	B	5–1–81	

The process of developing performance objectives is relatively simple, although at first it will seem lengthy. The time is worth it!

1. Brainstorm out job duties with individual staff members. Develop these into operationalized objectives.
2. Ask staff to rate objectives with regards to percentage of the total time the objective takes to accomplish.
3. *Negotiate* final percentage and specifics of each objective (e.g., rate, numbers).
4. Determine authority.
5. *Negotiate* due date and date for performance review.

Applying Learning Principles to Staff

Periodic performance evaluation will often point to areas of job-related behaviors that staff need to increase, decrease, or maintain. The principles of learning discussed in previous chapters apply to staff as well as to clients. Given what you now know about performance objectives and what motivates staff (see the section below on motivation, which gives some clues as to the broad classes of reinforcers for staff), it should be possible to directly initiate programs that positively change staff behavior. We suggest that, after the specific behavior you wish to affect has been operationalized and communicated to the staff person, the following guidelines be utilized:

1. *Involve staff in program decisions*—Remember, commitment directly follows from a person's involvement in the decision-making process.
2. *Assess staff skills*—If you expect staff to engage in a particular behavior (e.g., maintaining an adequate client data base, writing sound objectives), it is necessary to determine whether staff have the necessary skills. Skill development is not necessarily related to how long the person has been employed, or to his or her educational history. If staff do not have the necessary skills, in-service training might be a prerequisite to any change program.
3. *Provide frequent feedback*—Try to catch your staff doing things right. Frequent feedback regarding the correctness (or incorrectness) of behavior is a critical component of successful behavior change. Remember, it is highly likely that you think you give more positive feedback to staff than they perceive you giving.
4. *Teach staff to provide self-feedback*—Charting, graphing, and other self-monitoring techniques (see Chapter 14) can be powerful reminders to staff of particular behaviors they need to change.
5. *Teach staff to reinforce each other*—Openness in communication is positively related to organizational health. Encourage and model interpersonal reinforcement.
6. *Avoid burnout*—Become familiar with symptoms of staff burnout, such as high rates of illness, absenteeism, negative thinking (statements of despair: "Yes but . . .", "We tried that!"), or rigidity ("It won't work here"). Clear job expectations and reinforcement for a job "well done" and a feeling of control over one's life can reduce burnout. Additionally, we encourage staff to space vacation days (as opposed to taking block time) and encourage "mental health" days. For an excellent discussion of staff burnout see Greenberg and Valletutti (1980).

SHARED NEEDS

Kaiser (1975) has suggested that antiquated concepts have created organizations with "unclear missions, staffed by unknowledgeable people producing indeterminant products for unknown constituencies'' (p. 3). One possible solution to this problem is to intentionally design the organization to maximize the shared needs of people and programs [see Schein (1978) for an excellent book on matching individual and organizational needs]. Kaiser (1975) presented the following ecosystem design process for organizations whose primary role is caring for other people.

Stage 1—The development of organizational values. The primary role of community-based programs for developmentally disabled persons is to provide habilitative programming. However, this value may not be shared by staff, funding agencies, or significant others in the client's life. Critical to the success of the organization is that the values of the ecosystem, that is, the organization and the environment in which it operates, be brought into congruence. We all can think of instances where the organization had one goal (e.g., placement of the client in competitive employment) and significant others had differing values for the client (e.g., placement in a sheltered setting). Unless values are shared the system will continue to work at cross purposes.

Stage 2—Values are translated into specific goals. Although a program may have many possible values, certain ones are given a high-priority designation. These are then selected for implementation. By establishing shared values, the probability that all members of the system will have commitment to the implementation of the values is increased.

Stage 3—Methodology for achievement of goals is established. Just as with the client, when we have decided where we are and where we are going, there may be a variety of different methodologies to achieve organizational goals. It is particularly important to look at the range and scope of the ecosystem in which the program operates. For example, if the program is committed to increasing client independence, the program will have to work with parents, the business community, state agencies, and possibly the legislature, as well as in-house staff. Methodology for achieving a goal of increased client independence would be different for each one of these groups. Thus, there will not be a unidimensional methodology for any goal. Methodology will have to be individualized to meet the needs of the particular component of the ecosystem.

Stage 4—Programs must be matched to staff and clients' needs. Once goals and methods are clearly operationalized it becomes evident that not all staff and not all clients are able to benefit or work effectively in all environments. Because of the range of individual differences, it is important that there be a "goodness of fit" between people and programs.

Stage 5—The staff's perception of the program environment is measured and compared with goals of the program. This is a mapping process. If both staff and client are to benefit from a planned environment, clearly they must be able to perceive and utilize the available resources.

Stage 6—The staff's behavior in the environment is monitored and compared with their perception of that environment and the goals of the environment. All three—goals, perception, and behavior—should be in correspondence.

Stage 7—All of the data collected throughout the system is fed back to Stage 1, where new values may be selected or old values that have failed to achieve success through the process may be redesigned.

If the administrator is developing a new program he or she may begin at Stage 1 and continue on to Stage 7 in a stepwise fashion. However, if the program is already in existence and the administrator wishes to implement planned organizational change, he or she may begin with Stage 5—that is, the mapping stage—and proceed through to Stage 7 (Kaiser, 1975).

MOTIVATION

Much has been written about what motivates staff, and no approach to the management, development, and continued productivity of any organization would be complete without some discussion about motivation. Much of the success or failure of any program is dependent upon the motivation of the staff.

Exercise

15-1. What's your theory of motivation? The following questionnaire was developed by Bill Garove and Tom Fernekes of the Management Training Program at the University of Alabama, Birmingham. Mark the statements as A for agree, or DA for disagree. Go back over the statements after completing this section on motivation, and note any changes.

1. A strict enforcement of all rules and regulations is the only effective way to increase output from most workers.
2. The surest way to encourage a worker's maximum contribution is to offer financial rewards for doing more.
3. Most employees prefer a job that requires very little thought.
4. Most employees try harder to carry out decisions if they have a hand in making the decisions that affect them.
5. For most employees what they do is not as important as what they earn.
6. High employee morale is the best assurance of maximum worker effort and contribution.
7. Only a few employees can contribute creatively in work; the rest must always be told in detail what to do.
8. Good working conditions ensure high levels of worker output.
9. Personal conscience cannot assure a fair day's work from most workers. Performance standards must be rigidly enforced.
10. Fear is always an effective motivator.

Herzberg (1966) developed a concept referred to as the motivation-hygiene theory from a study of 200 engineers and accountants. He was able to identify two discrete types of events: those that led to job satisfaction and increased productivity (motivation) and those that produced job dissatisfaction (hygiene). Motivators were those factors that increased satisfaction and productivity. Top-rated motivators were achievement, recognition for achievement, the nature of work itself, responsibility, and potential for advancement.

Hygiene factors were related to job dissatisfaction. That is, there was a minimal maintenance level, and any deficits in this produced dissatisfaction. Hygiene factors include: company policy and administration, supervision, salary, interpersonal relations, and working conditions.

Given this distinction between motivators and hygiene factors, it is possible to have an unmotivated employee who isn't dissatisfied, or a motivated employee who is dissatisfied. An important point to note is that hygiene factors are not to be confused with motivators, and that their motivation effects, if any, are short term (Herzberg, 1968).

For example, we often complain about the lack of salary money for staff in our developmental disabilities programs. Although we should not dismiss its importance as a hygiene factor, we should not consider it as a motivator. Herzberg (1968) suggests that money motivates staff to seek the next pay increase, but is not necessarily related to increased satisfaction and productivity.

Achievement, recognition, challenging work, and responsibility are factors that produce productive and satisfied employees. But how often do these things occur in an organization? One thing we do know is that supervisors and employees differ considerably in their perceptions of how frequently these events occur. Table 15-1 (Likert, 1961) shows a distinct discrepancy.

Table 15-1. Differences in supervisor and employee perceptions[a]

	Supervisors: How do you reward good work? (% of supervisors who say "very often")	Employees: How does your supervisor reward good work? (% of employees who said "very often")
Gives privileges	52	14
Gives more responsibility	48	10
Gives a pat-on-the-back	82	13
Gives sincere praise	80	14
Gives more interesting work	51	5

[a] Data from: Likert, R. *New patterns of management.* New York: McGraw-Hill, 1961.

Abraham Maslow (1954) presents a slightly different picture of motivation, although both he and Herzberg view personal achievement as a high form of motivation. The basic premise of Maslow's theory of motivation is that people have an internal drive toward self-fulfillment. However, higher-order needs are effective as motivators only when certain basic needs have been achieved. Thus, Maslow believes that motivation comes from within the person.

In developing the Hierarchy of Needs, Maslow (1954) identified the following five levels of need:

1. *Physiological*—These needs are on the lowest level and have to do with the maintenance of physical comfort.
2. *Safety*—This involves the elimination of the threat of physical or emotional harm to the individual.
3. *Social*—Where the first two levels of need concern primarily the individual alone, this level relates to the need to interact and belong to some social group.
4. *Esteem*—This involves not only respect from others, but self-respect as well. People need to have positive feelings about who they are and what they do.
5. *Self-actualization*—This is the highest level need. Self-actualization means achievement of a person's full potential.

In applying Maslow's theory to the organization, a manager must be perceptive of the level of need for a particular employee. Thus, a given individual might only wish to survive (a 1/1 manager?) in the organization (thus satisfying his or her physiological and safety needs), and offering this employee creativity and esteem would not be likely to lead to high production.

Herzberg (1968) suggests the following steps to establishing motivators for employees:

1. Select those jobs in which costs do not make changes prohibitive, attitudes are poor, hygiene is costly, and motivation could make a difference.
2. Approach these jobs with the belief that there is another way to do things.
3. Brainstorm a list of changes, without regard to practicality.
4. Screen to eliminate suggestions that involve hygiene factors.
5. Make certain suggestions are well defined and operationalized.
6. Prioritize the suggestions.
7. Implement the suggestions.
8. Provide feedback to employees regarding productivity before and after implementation.

ORGANIZATIONAL MAKE-UP

Too often, organizations seem to run on the personalities involved. Although this can facilitate organizational functioning if all parties are skilled, benign, and helpful, it can be devastating if the people change. Furthermore, it can be highly destructive if the personalities are inconsistent. Thus, all organizations need to be concerned with long-term structure with regard to how things work.

A Table of Organization (TO) is a schematic representation of the *structure, authority,* and *communication* within the organization. It is the document that shows graphically how the organization should communicate. A first step in developing a cohesive organization is the development of a TO that reflects the functions of the organization.

In developing a TO for your organization, Scheerenberger (1975) suggests utilizing one of the following models (see Figure 15-1):

Traditional Medical   The medical model divides the organization into three units: clinical, specialized services, and business or financial. The clinical services division is responsible for all program services, and specialized services included all "non-medical" specialties. This model is widely adopted, and no longer limited to medical models. For example, in many special education programs, the teacher(s) fill the role of clinical services. The problem with this organizational model is that the components do not interact in any organized fashion.

Traditional Non-medical   The non-medical model was developed in reaction to the medical model (Roselle, 1952). In this TO, the organization is structured more along discipline or functional lines. There are numerous consequences for this type of TO, including a tendency to treat the client in a piecemeal fashion and the lack of interaction between units. The main reason for changing from a medical to non-medical model would be an attempt to "divide and conquer" by a director.

Standard Unit   This TO attempts to combine a variety of personnel into autonomously functioning units. The rationale behind the unit approach is based on the functional grouping of clients into services components (units). Thus, staff are not divided along disciplinary lines, but along their interactive patterns with clients. One problem with this approach is that, in the construction of the TO, particular attention must be given to communication/decision-making authority within the agency, as well as to unit functioning.

Quasi-unit   The basic difference between the quasi-unit and the standard unit approach is that the quasi-unit TO takes into account the fact that, although staff may be assigned to a given unit or project, departmental or professional affiliations may still exist within the program. With this approach, unless authority and decision-making powers are clearly spelled out, staff may be torn between the unit director and a departmental affiliation.

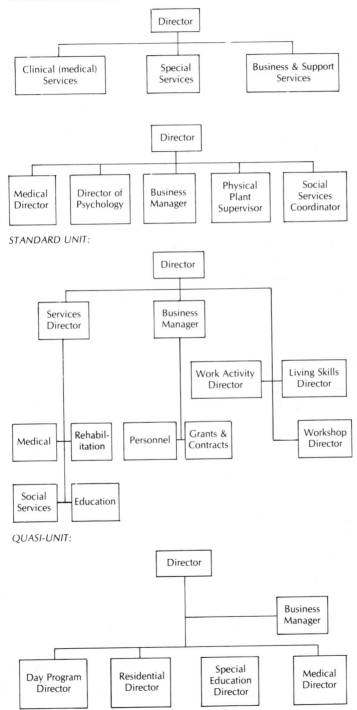

TRADITIONAL MEDICAL:

STANDARD UNIT:

QUASI-UNIT:

Figure 15-1. Four types of Tables of Organization. (Adapted from Scheerenberger, 1975.)

287

In summary, a Table of Organization that accurately reflects lines of authority and decision-making—and is followed in practice—helps staff to know who is responsible and whom to approach with problems.

FREE EXPRESSION OF IDEAS

It should be evident from discussions in both this chapter and Chapter 14 that the organization that encourages the free expression of ideas gets both better ideas and commitment by staff to those ideas.

PROVISION OF FEEDBACK

Objectivity and mutually agreed upon goals can serve to reduce much of the threat of performance evaluation sessions. However, if a manager is to effectively influence a staff person, he or she must have an awareness of his or her impact on that person. Go back and review the communication models and problems presented in the previous chapter. Remember that the major goals of the performance feedback sessions are to:

1. Reinforce appropriate behaviors.
2. Provide corrective feedback.
3. Assist individuals to achieve their full potential.
4. Provide staff with an opportunity to see themselves as perceived by another person.

Levinson (1962) has identified four barriers to fully developing staff skills within performance evaluation sessions:

1. *Lack of time*—Extensive interaction and performance appraisal is often limited to an annual basis. More frequent interaction is necessary to produce change.
2. *No mistakes allowed*—Much like the proactive staff, a proactive manager must look for and emphasize the positive aspects of employee performance. Focusing on the mistakes leads to a lack of creativity on the part of employees. People are so "gun-shy" that they are afraid to take a risk that might lead to a creative or a poor decision.
3. *Rivalry is repressed*—Many superiors are afraid of being "dethroned" by subordinates. This type of manager rarely hires (for very long) any subordinate who might, in any way, exceed the superior's abilities.
4. *Superior-subordinate relationship is unexamined*—In America we are particularly uncomfortable with the realities of power and status. This

tends to result in one-way communication. Communication must be a two-way street if the manager hopes to effectively influence employee performance.

COMMITMENT

Commitment to goals comes when people have a vested personal interest in the achievement of the goals. Kaiser's (1975) steps outlined earlier are designed to encourage the development of shared goals. This is essential to developing staff commitment.

PLANNED CHANGE IN ORGANIZATIONAL DEVELOPMENT

We suggest that the following steps be utilized in any planned change for an organization:

1. Education
2. Team building
3. Intergroup problem-solving
4. Goal setting
5. Implementation

The first step in the organizational development process is education—in particular, education in the theories and uses of the managerial grid described in Chapter 15. If employees are given a frame of reference for managerial or supervisory behavior, they are then able to reinforce good and appropriate managerial behavior in each other. The second step is team building. Initially, this focuses on identifying and rectifying those problems that keep the group from most effectively functioning. Poor communication skills, lack of shared goals, and authority or hierarchical problems are only a few of the barriers to effective teamwork. Blake and Mouton (1964) suggest that team building have as its goals: 1) replace outmoded practices with a "team culture," 2) set standards of excellence, 3) increase personal objectivity, 4) utilize feedback to learn, and 5) establish objectives for team and individual achievement.

The third step in organizational development is intergroup problem-solving. During this step, different teams or groups are brought together for the purpose of achieving closer integration and resolving intergroup conflicts over such things as overlapping responsibility or fuzzy lines of authority. This is an important and critical phase for the community-based program for the developmentally disabled. Communication among various groups is often a source of trouble. Individual staff or managers in component groups of the organization oftentimes see only their group and fail to see their group as it relates to the whole organizational functioning. When such groups become isolated from the whole, intergroup rivalry increases and win/lose situations occur within the organization. The underlying problems of intergroup relationships must be dealt with before organizational development is attempted.

The next step in organizational development is goal setting and planning. The key to goal setting and planning is for the organization to have a clear sense of mission or purpose and be able to objectively compare through data-oriented feedback this model with what the organization currently is or has been. A total organization—that is, all groups from within the system—are brought together for target setting, the establishment of mutual commitment, and formulation of formal review procedures.

The fifth phase of organizational development is implementing the plan. Blake and Mouton (1964) compared this favorably to the remodeling of a building. When the architects and engineers study the existing structure, they identify what is strong, sound, and consistent with the proposed change and what parts of the building can be retained and incorporated. What is antiquated or inconsistent with the proposed change must either be replaced or modified or strengthened in order to make it consistent with the new goals. Once these decisions have been reached the carpenters and electricians know exactly what must be done in order to move from the old to the new.

SUGGESTED ACTIVITIES

1. For the next week ask three or four staff members from several levels of your organization to keep track of who they go to when they have a problem or need a decision. Then meet with these persons and compare their records to your TO. What differences did you find?
2. Develop performance objectives for your job.

ADDITIONAL RESOURCES

Blake, R., & Mouton, J. *Grid organizational development*. Houston: Gulf Publishing Co., 1968.
   The logical extension of the grid approach: how to apply the principles to organizational development.
Duncan, J. W. *Organizational behavior*. Boston: Houghton Mifflin Co., 1978.
   This clearly written book is a real how-to-do-it.

AUDIOVISUAL MATERIALS

Productivity and the self-fulfilling prophecy: The Pygmalion effect. Delmar, Calif.: CRM Productions, McGraw-Hill Films 1974.
   Do you believe that your expectations alone can have an effect on employee behavior? Do you believe that you have to even be aware of your expectations? See this film for startling answers.

REFERENCES

Bennis, W. G. *Organization development: Its nature, origins, and prospects.* Reading, Mass.: Addison-Wesley Publishing Co., 1969.

Blake, R. R., & Mouton, J. S. *The managerial grid.* Houston: Gulf Publishing Co., 1964.

Boyd, B. B., & Jensen, J. M. Perceptions of the first line supervisor's authority: A study of superior subordinate communication. *Academy of Management Journal,* 1972, *15,* 331–342.

Burke, R. J., & Wilcox, D. S. Characteristics of effective emphasis performance review and development interviews. *Personnel Psychology,* 1969, *22,* 219–305.

French, W. Organization development: Objectives, assumptions, and strategies. *California Management Review,* 1969, *12*(2), 26.

Greenberg, S. F., & Valletutti, P. J. *Stress and the helping professions.* Baltimore: Paul H. Brookes Publishers, 1980.

Greene, C. N. Relationships among role accuracy compliance, performance evaluation, and satisfaction within managerial dyads. *Academy of Management Journal,* 1972, *15,* 205–216.

Hamerlynck, L. A. When you pass the behavioral buck—make it contingent, or reflection upon service in state government. *The Behavior Therapist,* 1980, *3*(5), 5–9.

Herzberg, F. *Work and the nature of man.* Cleveland: World Publishing Co., 1966.

Herzberg, F. One more time: How do you motivate employees. *Harvard Business Review,* January-February 1968, pp. 53–62.

Kaiser, L. R. *The ecosystem model: Designing organizational environments.* Presented at the Annual Meeting of the Society for General Systems Research, New York, January 27–30, 1975.

Levinson, D. J. A psychologist looks at executive development. *Harvard Business Review,* 1962, *40,* 69–75.

Likert, R. *New patterns of management.* New York: McGraw-Hill, 1961.

Maslow, A. H. *Motivation and personality.* New York: Harper & Row, 1954.

Miner, J. B. *Personnel psychology.* New York: Macmillan, 1969.

Roselle, E. Some thoughts on the administrative organization of a training school for mental defectives. *American Journal on Mental Deficiency,* 1952, *56*(3), 524–536.

Scheerenberger, R. C. *Managing residential facilities for the developmentally disabled.* Springfield, Ill.: Charles C Thomas, 1975.

Schein, E. H. *Career dynamics: Matching individual and organizational needs.* Reading, Mass.: Addison-Wesley, 1978.

Triandis, H. C. Differential perceptions of certain jobs and people by managers, clerks, and workers in industry. *Journal of Applied Psychology,* 1959, *43,* 221–225.

Triandis, H. C. Cognitive similarity and communication in a dyad. *Human Relations,* 1960, *13,* 175–183.

Chapter 16

Effective Case Management

OBJECTIVES

To be able to:

1. Define case management.
2. Describe four responsibilities of a case manager.
3. Describe the relationship between case management and client advocacy.
4. Write in SOAP format:
   a. Report to file (e.g., case conference).
   b. Note to file (e.g., critical incident).

How many of these statements collected by us from community-based programs in over 10 states have you heard?

> "Hey, anybody seen Mary Smith's file?"
>
> "Weren't you supposed to call his parents?"
>
> "There was nothing we could do. Dr. Moore wouldn't tell why he increased the meds."
>
> "I don't know why she's placed here."
>
> "Her parents never bring her when it rains."
>
> "Well, whose responsibility is it anyway? The production manager usually overrules client placement."

It is the activities involved in case management that are the final key to providing proactive habilitation services for clients. Acting as primary coordinator, the case manager must synchronize all the different services needed to provide the best programming for an individual client. Although individual states, or regions within states, may have their own definition of case management, we define case management in a rather unique way. Case management is the *process* by which responsibility for implementation and evaluation of the client's program plan is established. It is important to note that case management is a process. This process includes providing support, processing direct services, coordinating services, collecting and disseminating data, and monitoring the progress of the client.

TASKS OF THE CASE MANAGER

More specifically, we view the following seven activities as the tasks of a case manager.

1. The case manager attends to the total spectrum of client needs—including housing, family relationships, financial matters, health, education, program records, and training needs—regardless of whether these services are provided by the agency.

2. The case manager provides supportive services to the client and the client's family. This includes correcting misunderstandings and encouraging participation by significant others where appropriate in client programs. All case managers *must* be completely familiar with the legal obligations described in Chapter 2, as well as the federal (PL 94-142) and state regulations outlined in detail in Chapters 4 and 5. Many parents and significant others misunderstand their legal relationship with the client, and the case manager must act as an information source for parents and clients. For example, many parents simply assume they are the client's guardian "just because the client is retarded." However, guardianship is a *legal* decision after the client reaches the age of majority (18–21 in most states). Unless guardianship has been legally determined by a court, the client is his or her own guardian. We encourage all case managers to establish a working relationship with the state's legal advocacy program. Contact your state office of developmental disabilities for information regarding your state's protection and advocacy (P & A) program.

3. The case manager locates and procures services outside the agency when needed. This relates back to one of the original characteristics of a proactive staff person: know the agency. In addition, the proactive case manager must effectively advocate for services that the client needs, but which the agency can't or doesn't provide.

4. The case manager coordinates the delivery of all services to the client. The case manager is responsible for scheduling and determining priorities. You will soon discover, if you have not already, that every component (e.g., vocational, residential, educational) of the habilitation team has a tendency to consider what they offer to be most important. It is the case manager's job to determine priorities and avoid fights over "ownership" of the client.

5. The case manager secures all relevant data and information from other agencies in order to keep the program plan up to date. One instance in which programming often breaks down is when a client is receiving services outside

the agency. Oftentimes staff do not seem to know what's happening at the residential program, what's happening in counseling or why the client's medication was suddenly decreased. It is the responsibility of the case manager to coordinate and disseminate relevant data and information from all service delivery components.

6. The case manager monitors the operation of services that are provided to the client. This is truly where the *process* of advocacy for the client comes in. The case manager must be aware of what are "quality" services, and what can be done to improve services that are deficient. Additionally, the appropriateness of services delivered must be constantly evaluated.

Let's tune in on the following discussion overheard in a case conference:

Staff 1:   "Look, I'm convinced that the new furniture stripping program will be just the thing to keep Bill busy."
Staff 2:   "But he's severely retarded, non-verbal, and seems to me to need some pretty specific kinds of social skill training."
Staff 1:   "But you know how dependent he gets. Individual attention just spoils him. Besides, he's gotta learn to work sometime."
Parent: "I'm sure you'll do the best for Billy. Just remember how scared he gets when he has to leave here for anything."
Staff 2:   "But that's just the point, Mr. Jones..."
Staff 1:   (interrupting) "Don't worry Mr. Jones, we'll make sure Billy's well taken care of."

As case manager what would you do, and how would you go about doing it? The case manager's *first* responsibility is to the client. Unless this is understood by staff and administration alike, problems are bound to occur.

7. A case manager provides documentation relative to the review of the client's IPP. Many types of data collection procedures were described in Chapter 6. An additional form of monitoring that we recommend be implemented is what is known as the Problem-Oriented Record.

PROBLEM-ORIENTED RECORD

The Problem-Oriented Record (POR) was originally developed as the Problem-Oriented Medical Record (POMR) (Weed, 1968a, b). The POR provides a logical, systematic, and orderly way to record case notes or notes to the client's file. There are four components to the POR.

1. Data Base—"What Do We Know About the Client?"

The data base is the basic information used in identifying a client's problems and developing the individual program plan. It would include:

1. Client history
2. Medical evaluations, diagnosis
3. Psychological evaluation

4. Education and vocational test reports
5. Adaptive behavior scales
6. Data collection
7. Educational, vocational, and behavior treatment plans

2. Problem List—"What Are the Problems?"

1. Definition—A problem is any identifiable fact that may have a significant influence on the client's health and quality of life. A problem may include items of case management, medical, psychological, educational, vocational, social, or behavioral significance. For example:

   Many clients have a significant weight problem. In society today, this can have far-reaching effects on the client socially, vocationally, avocationally, and medically. A significant weight problem can influence the client's acceptance in the community and the types of jobs and leisure activities the client can engage in, and may pose a risk to the cardiovascular system. Weight would, in this case, rank as a problem along with others such as living situation or employability.

2. Construction of the problem list—It is the responsibility of the staff to identify the client problems and enter them on the Client Problem List by using consecutive numbers and titles (see Table 16-1). Each problem is assigned a number and title by which it is subsequently identified throughout the records. All problems listed must be dated as to when the problem was first noted by staff. A SOAP (see below) will be completed by a staff member at that time. The Problem List is always the first page of the client's active and master file.

3. Entering of additional problems—After the initial problem list is created, new problems will arise as the client participates in the program. Each new problem is dated and recorded under a new number of the problem list. It is necessary that adequate documentation be made in the record to substantiate the problem. Each problem added to the problem list should have in the progress note section a dated note including the number, title, and the SOAP formula. Furthermore, each problem is noted as "A" for active (meaning still occurring) or "IA" for inactive.

4. Temporary problems—Minor episodes may arise in the course of a client's care that may not be of enough significance to place on the problem list. Here the progress note may be titled as a temporary problem, followed by the appropriate SOAP format. If such a temporary problem persists, a decision must be made as to whether to add it to the problem list or to drop it as being insignificant. For example, a single or even a couple of emotional outbursts would probably not be added to a problem list. Similarly, an incident of theft, an argument, or unhappiness would likely not qualify as a problem. However, if these incidents occurred frequently, or on a regular basis, they would become problems.

Table 16-1. Problem list

NAME: __Joe Campell_____ DATE: _Feb. 20, 1979____
AGE: __25_____ SEX: __Male_____

Problem number	Problem	Date	Active/ inactive	Treatment Plan	Review
8	Seizures	2/1/79	A	Monitor present medication—Judith	2/28/79
40	Physical aggression	2/1/79	A	Behavioral tr. plan—collect data—Pat	2/7/79
33	Reading—Functional word recognition	2/1/79	A	Educ. prog.—Word recogn. Man, women, exit, entrance—Pat	4/30/79
2	Funding—Title XX eligibility	2/1/79	A	Complete necessary forms; renew reg. for eligibility—Marty	4/30/79
23	Leisure skills—Client needs a skill to participate in community activity	2/1/79	A	Initiate bowling program—Alice	4/30/79
30	On-job training—Need assist sweeping	2/1/79	A	T/A sweeping; steps 1–12—Brian	4/30/79

5. Revision of problem list—When several problems turn out to be separate manifestations of a single problem, then these problems should be grouped together and given a new number. In this instance all previous numbers are dropped. For example, suppose the client's problem list included (3) rapid eye movements, (4) dizziness, and (5) blackouts. After further study the client is diagnosed as having seizures. The new listing would be:

> Problem #8: Seizures
> a) Rapid eye movements
> b) Dizziness
> c) Blackouts—2–3 minutes

Problem lists should be reviewed and updated as indicated when new supporting data are acquired. Again, each problem will have its own identification number, which will be consistent throughout the records.

3. Plan—"What Am I Going to Do?"

For each identified problem, staff will list the appropriate treatment strategies. These can include a list of additional diagnostic or supportive information and specific educational or behavioral treatment strategies. For example:

Problem	Date	Plan	Review
1. Seizures	2/1/79	Appt. w/physician for medication—Jo	2/6/79
2. Self-injurious behavior—head banging	2/8/79	Collect baseline data when behavior occurs. Behavioral Treatment Plan to extinguish S.I.B.—Pat	2/18/79

4. Progress Notes—"How Are We Doing?"

Definition The progress notes coordinate with the problem list and the plan. They reflect new or changing behaviors, additional evaluative information, the status and results of the program plan, responses of the client, reassessment of the problem, and new plans (Table 16-2).

Format Each progress note should include: the number of the problem, title, date, and the signature and title of person completing the note. The progress note will be completed utilizing the SOAP format.

Subjective—Contains data from the client's point of view. Client statements.
Objective—Significant data that are compiled or gathered on a client. Would include: test results, evaluation reports.
Assessment—Discussion, analysis of the objective/subjective data or treatment.
Plan—Treatment or intervention strategies utilized.

The SOAP note should be entered as frequently as necessary to document significant events. It is recommended that SOAP notes be completed at least once a week. *New* problems should be evaluated in the progress notes and should be added to the problem list as noted in the Problem Section.

SUGGESTED ACTIVITIES

1. Take an available client file and:
   a. Conduct staffing.
   b. Gather data base.
   c. Complete problem list.
   d. Do initial SOAP on each problem.
2. Take three client treatment programs that you have developed and SOAP the client's current progress.

Table 16-2. Progress Notes

NAME: ___Joe Campbell___ COMPLETED BY: _____
TITLE: _____

Problem number	Problem	Date	
8	Seizures	2/7/79	S. Joe stated that he doesn't feel dizzy, and has not fainted in 2 days. O. Joe has been actively engaged in all tasks, and has not displayed seizure activity at Center. A. Medication seems to work. P. Continue to monitor Joe and medication.
40	Physical aggression	2/7/79	S. "No, I will not," Joe stated. O. Joe would not complete task, and struck trainer. A. Joe frustrated with task, unable to control anger. P. Simplify task for success; utilize timeout when he initially becomes angry.
33	Reading—Functional word	2/7/79	O. After showing flash card and stating word, Joe is able to repeat it without error 100% time. A. Methodology seems to work, he stays on task. P. Continue program.
2	Funding—Title XX	2/5/79	S. Joe stated "I want to stay here—." O. Joe has improved in voc. skills, funct. academics, and community living skills since he has been enrolled. He is now 21 and ineligible for Spec. Ed. funds. P. Check county of residence to see if Joe will be eligible for Title XX at this facility.

(continued)

Table 16-2. (*continued*)

Problem number	Problem	Date	
23	Leisure—Bowling	2/8/79	S. Joe says he likes to go bowling. O. Joe is unable to coordinate walk and roll ball—ball goes into gutter. A. Need to simplify task, concentrate on one aspect of skill. P. Joe will stand at line and roll ball, we'll provide physical guidance.
30	Job training—Sweep	2/9/79	O. After being told "Joe, sweep the floor," Joe goes through steps 1–4 independently. A. Program working well, Joe enjoys task. P. Continue w/ task analysis. Concentrate on steps 5–7.

Key: S = subjective; O = objective; A = assessment; P = plan.

ADDITIONAL RESOURCES

Problem oriented medical record—Procedures manual. Jamestown, N.D.: Dakota State Hospital, August 1976.

Rybock, R., & Gardner, J. Problem formulation: The problem oriented record. *American Journal of Psychiatry,* 1973, 130(3), 312-316.

REFERENCES

Weed, L. L. Medical records that guide and teach. *The New England Journal of Medicine,* March 14, 1968, *278,* 593.

Weed, L. L. Medical records that guide and teach. *The New England Journal of Medicine,* March 21, 1968, *278,* 652-657.

Resource Utilization
Traveler's Aid

Chapter 17

Professional, Community, and Information Resources

OBJECTIVES

To be able to:

1. List the reason for using professional resources.
2. List information you need to give to professionals.
3. List information needed from professionals.
4. List different types of professional resources that may be needed by your clients.
5. Identify at least four reasons for using community resources.
6. Identify community resources that may meet unfulfilled client needs.
7. Identify relevant professional organizations and what they can do for you.
8. Contact these organizations for more information or membership applications.
9. Identify relevant professional journals and subscribe to them.
10. Contact and use other information resources such as libraries, technical resource centers, computerized data bases, university-affiliated facilities, and federal agencies to obtain professional information.

The reason that your agency should utilize professional, community, and information resources is that one agency cannot possibly be all things to all people. In other words, your agency cannot be expected to and should not try to serve every client's every need. Remember, proactive staff know which needs their agency can serve and which ones it cannot serve. Usually one of two things happens to agencies that try to take care of everything for everyone: either they end up providing inadequate services for everyone or else they provide services that are not really needed. That is, very often services rendered are not necessarily services needed. A client is provided with a service simply because that is the service the agency happens to provide, not because it is one that the client really needs. Also, services provided are sometimes not necessarily those wanted. For instance, individuals who want to be food service workers may find themselves in a janitorial training program because the agency serving them does not have the facilities or staff to train food service workers but does have a janitorial training program. If your agency does not provide a service that a client needs or wants, try to find that service in your community.

PROFESSIONAL RESOURCES

When you decide to consult an outside professional, you must carefully consider what information you need to provide to the professional and what information you should request from the professional both before and after this individual has seen your client. We look on the consulting of professional resources as sort of a smaller version of the goal-planning process: in order to get the best results, you need to know where you want to go. You need to have a clearly developed reason for consulting that individual. In other words, what will your client get out of the consultation? All professionals find consultation easier when they know what is expected of them.

Giving Information

The first major consideration when you decide to consult an outside professional is: what information must you give that individual about your client's needs? The general rule of thumb here should be, as we have emphasized throughout this book, to be as specific and operational as possible when providing information. When considering what information you will take to a professional you are consulting, use the same kind of approach you would take if you were consulting that person for yourself. Remember, because many of your clients are not able to speak for themselves, you must speak for them during a professional consultation.

The most obvious type of information you will need to provide is the reason that you chose to consult a professional at this time. For example, if you are consulting a physician you will need to give a clear description of whatever medical symptoms have led you to approach this individual. Information regarding other medical treatment your client is currently receiving is also important when you consult a physician, particularly information about medication. You should also have information available regarding what types of services your client has received in the past from the type of professional you are consulting. Additionally, be prepared to provide a description of all of the different types of services your client is currently receiving.

Getting Information

There are two types of information you need to obtain from the professional you consult. The first type is information that you need to obtain prior to actually making an appointment for your client. Specifically, you need to find out what types of services this particular professional provides. For example, not all psychologists provide all of the different types of psychological services that are available. Psychologists specialize in particular kinds of therapy or particular kinds of approaches to assessment. That information is extremely important for you to have before deciding whether you want to pursue contact with the professional. It would also be extremely helpful to inquire as to whether the individual professional you are consulting has had any previous experience working with developmentally disabled individuals and/or is willing to work with them.

The second type of information that you need to obtain from professionals you consult is what is recommended for your client. This includes services the professional can provide and services which he or she can teach you to provide. We say teach you to provide because a speech therapist, for example, may be able to teach you how to supplement speech therapy by having your client do certain communication exercises throughout the day. A neurologist may be able to teach you to identify seizures that require immediate medical attention, what to do during seizures, and how to recognize situations in which a client is pretending to have a seizure. These types of situations are examples of the reason that we say you should ask both what services the client is going to receive and what services the professional might be able to teach you to provide.

Regardless of what any particular professional recommends for your client, we recommend that you obtain in writing a description of both the recommendations made for your client and the reasons why those particular recommendations were made. This information should become a part of your client's permanent records. When you get recommendations in writing, everyone involved with your client can read them and thus receive information directly from the consultant. This tends to be more accurate than passing information on verbally. Furthermore, written recommendations serve as proof of what service your client received and why.

Professional Services That May Be Useful

Medical Services   In addition to the general medical services we all need, your clients will probably at some point need to consult a variety of medical specialists. The list of the different types of medical specialties is extremely lengthy and we have no intention of providing a comprehensive one here. However, we do want to point out several of the specialties that are most likely to be needed by your clients.

A neurologist is a physician who has special training in dealing with disorders of the brain and nervous system, such as epilepsy. Any of your clients who are regularly receiving medication for control of epileptic seizures should be consulting a neurologist on a regular basis. A psychiatrist is a physician who is primarily concerned with emotional/behavioral disorders. Consultation with a psychiatrist is extremely important whenever you have a client who is receiving psychotropic medications. This is because psychiatrists are the only physicians who have received extensive training in the use of these types of medications and their effect on behavior.

An internist is a physician who has received postgraduate training in the diagnosis and treatment of adults by nonsurgical means. Some internists have also received additional training in more specialized areas such as cardiology (which involves diseases of the heart and blood vessels). A gynecologist is a physician who is trained in the treatment of the female organs. All of your female clients over the age of 18 should be seeing a gynecologist for regular checkups. An ophthalmologist is specially trained in the treatment of diseases of the eye.

Another type of medical specialist we find that our clients often do not visit regularly and should is the dentist. Dentists specialize in the care of teeth and the gums, and in diseases of the mouth. Many developmentally disabled individuals have not received sufficient dental care to maintain healthy teeth and gums.

Health-Related Services   Probably the health-related services most often used by agencies serving the developmentally disabled are physical therapy, occupational therapy, and speech therapy. Physical therapists specialize in the use of various physical approaches to reducing pain and/or improving or maintaining physical functioning. Occupational therapists use a wide variety of activities designed to promote improved levels of sensorimotor functioning. Speech therapists provide diagnosis and therapy for speech and language problems. In addition you may at times find it useful to consult with your local public health nurse, a nutritionist, or a respiratory therapist.

Social Services   You are also probably used to having extensive contact with professionals who provide social services. Social workers are typically involved with the individuals you serve through state or federal welfare agencies. They often help your clients obtain financial assistance either directly or in the form of aid such as food stamps. They are also trained to work with family systems and usually have fairly extensive information about family situations. Vocational rehabilitation counselors are usually found in the local office of your state's division of vocational rehabilitation. They can assist your clients in obtaining support from the division of vocational rehabilitation for services such as job training and placement.

Psychologists   Psychologists can provide a variety of different services

to your clients. It is particularly important to rem
earlier about the fact that not all members of a prof/
services available from members of that profession.
chologists specialize in testing, others specialize in individua.
specialize in family therapy. Psychologists also vary greatly in terms
they approach human problems. It would be wise to get some idea of how a
particular psychologist approaches your client's problems in order to determine whether that individual's approach is consistent with the approach that is
taken by your agency.

Special Educators   Special educators are teachers who have been
trained to provide instruction to individuals with handicapping conditions or
learning difficulties. As with psychologists, special educators vary with respect to how they approach problems and particularly with respect to what age
and type of individual they are trained to serve. You will, of course, need to
work very closely with special educators regarding any of your clients who are
still receiving public school services. Perhaps the most important way in
which these individuals can be of assistance to you is in the area of curriculum
design and instructional techniques.

Advocates   The final category of professionals whom you may wish to
consult for your client is the advocate. There are a variety of types of advocates available to your clients. Perhaps the type with which we are most
familiar is the legal advocate, that is, the attorney. In addition, in many
communities there are what are called citizen advocates. Citizen advocates are
volunteers who defend the rights and interests of the client and provide practical or emotional reinforcement for him or her (National Association for Retarded Citizens, 1974).

Summary

These are some of the professional resources that may be of use to your
clients. There are undoubtedly others that we have neglected to mention. We
hope that we have included those you are most likely to use often. The
important point here is that you will need these resources because your agency
cannot be all things to all people.

COMMUNITY RESOURCES

We have identified at least four reasons that agencies providing direct services
should use community resources. The first of these relates to the ultimate goal
of service delivery. We believe that goal should be for clients to become
independent members of their communities. In order for someone to be a
member of his or her community, he or she needs to be integrated into that
community and to interact with the various components of it. As was noted in
Chapter 3 ("Community-Referenced Programming"), it is not enough for

meone to live in a community. Interaction with the various aspects of the community is also necessary, hence the need to use community resources.

The second reason we have identified for using community resources is to help select appropriate standards for programming. In other words, we need to attend to community standards when we set client goals. The reason for this is that what is acceptable in one community may be entirely different from what is acceptable in another community (Elder, 1980). That standards vary between different communities should be obvious when you stop to think about the differences in behavior between people on the sidewalks of New York and people on the farms of South Dakota. Although there are certainly differences between any two urban communities or between any two rural communities, the differences between rural and urban areas are even more apparent. These differences most often appear when people delivering services in rural areas face the problems of arranging for transportation and communication in rural communities.

In addition to being aware of differences between communities, we also need to be aware of differences within a community. One of the authors is familiar with a group of individuals who at one time lived in an institution on the edge of a wealthy subdivision of a small midwestern city. When these people walked through the streets of the wealthy subdivision they looked very out of place. However, several of the clients then moved to a group home located within two blocks of the downtown area in the same city. This area was populated with "shopping bag ladies" who picked through garbage, and a variety of other obviously deviant individuals. In the downtown setting, the clients who had looked so out of place in the wealthy suburb looked perfectly normal. In fact, if anything, they looked better than a lot of other people on the street.

As we look at differences among communities we also need to be aware of cultural differences that exist within a given community. Clearly, what is acceptable behavior to blacks is not necessarily acceptable to whites nor is it necessarily acceptable to American Indians. The important thing to remember about all of these differences is that, in selecting goals for an individual, you must attend to the behaviors that are accepted or required by the community in which the individual is going to live.

A third reason for using community resources is that it gives you an opportunity to educate people associated with community resources about those you serve and the services you provide. This reason for using your community is extremely important. Community-based programs are not likely to succeed without community acceptance (Gottlieb, 1975). There are at least three different kinds of education that you may be able to help provide. The first of these has to do with the dispelling of myths. Most of us are to some extent afraid of those things with which we are not familiar. Lack of familiarity with people who are disabled leads to myths such as all mentally retarded people are violent, all mentally retarded people are sex maniacs, or mental retardation is contagious. There is little known about the relationship between attitudes such as these and behavior toward retarded persons (Gottlieb, 1975). However, it seems unlikely that those who believe such myths will behave positively toward mentally retarded individuals. One caution: do not assume that simply exposing your community to those you serve will change community attitudes. There is evidence that this does not necessarily occur (Gottlieb, 1975). Instead, be prepared for the need to provide information about what you are doing and to demonstrate what your clients can do before you will achieve acceptance.

A second kind of education that you may help provide is education of professionals in your community, particularly professionals in private practice. Often professionals such as physicians who have been in practice for several years are not aware of current advances in service provision for individuals with handicaps (Elder, 1980). If you approach these individuals tactfully you may be able to help them become aware of new advances. The final type of education that you may be able to help provide is education of people who want to help your clients, but who see your agency as primarily custodial. That is, many people believe that the developmentally disabled, particularly the mentally retarded, are poor, helpless people who have to be taken care of like little children for the rest of their lives. When you try to overcome that belief it is important to remember that until very recently it *was* true that we did not know how to teach these people to become productive members of their communities. Therefore, the beliefs that you are trying to overcome were in the past very valid. Changing them is going to be a long shaping process.

The next reason for using community resources is very closely related to the educational reason. Use of those resources can help your agency to build community support for what you do. By support we mean money, people's time, and/or moral support. One of the things we have to remember when we try to build community support is that many times service agencies are seen by community members as being self-perpetuating and self-serving (Hall, 1980). Obviously agencies have some needs that are apart from the needs of the clients they serve. For instance, agencies need to pay their bills. Furthermore, most organizations try to meet both their needs and their clients' needs. The best way to avoid being seen by your community as an agency that is primarily interested in meeting its own needs is to avoid being that kind of agency. In other words, as long as you are meeting client needs and you can demonstrate that you are doing so, it is unlikely that your agency will be seen as strictly self-serving.

Using Community Resources

In order to use community resources you must first know what they are. The list we offer here is designed to give you ideas. It is by no means comprehensive and we are certain that you will find resources in your community that are not on this list. The list is simply intended to give you a place to start. Our list is adapted from one provided by Laten and Wikler (1978). They divided community resources into two types: formal and informal. Examples of formal resources are:

1. Church groups and clergy. This would include service groups run by churches, volunteer groups, and individual clergy.
2. Clubs or hobby groups. This might include your local YMCA or YWCA, biking clubs, hiking clubs, and so forth.
3. Service groups. This might include groups such as the Kiwanis, Shriners, Elks, Moose, and the Lions.
4. Businesses and business groups. This includes individual businesses, as well as business organizations such as the Chamber of Commerce.
5. Local government. This will include your local police department, library, fire department, etc.
6. Consumer groups. This includes not only local chapters of traditionally parent groups such as the Association for Retarded Citizens but also groups of people with handicaps, such as People First, that provide peer support groups.
7. Generic service agencies. There are a great many professional services that are available throughout this country that are not specifically designed to serve people with handicaps or disabilities but that serve those people as part of a larger group. These might include your city or county or state social services agency, local medical services, vocational training programs, educational programs, and legal or citizen advocacy programs.

The second type of community resource described by Laten and Wikler (1978) consists of informal resources. These include families, neighbors, and friends. When thinking of families we must not limit our thinking just to parents; often brothers and sisters and other relatives can be important resources for an individual. Perhaps the most difficult job that the direct service professional has is working with the families of the people they serve. All too often a great many misunderstandings and misconceptions are held by everyone who is part of this relationship.

The National Association for Retarded Citizens (NARC) has published a brief monograph entitled, *The Parent/Professional Partnership: How to Make it Work* (1977). We believe that what this monograph has to say can be useful not only in evaluating your relationships with parents and family members but also in evaluating your relationships with any other outside resources and the people who represent them. The monograph describes common ways in which professionals mishandle parents. These include assuming that parents are ignorant, behaving as if they know the solutions to all of their client's problems, treating parents as patients, not really listening to parents, not telling parents what is going on, and creating an atmosphere of hopelessness. The other side of the coin is that there are also common ways in which parents mishandle professionals. These include shopping around and therefore never giving one service agency a chance to prove whether it can help, unfair expectations for magically "curing" their child, dishonesty, unwillingness to listen, or unreasonable demands. Often these problems, as well as others that arise during relationships between agencies and outside resources, are the result of differing values about what is important. Differing values can lead to differing objectives and priorities for clients. Also, service providers and families or two different sets of service providers often put themselves in a position where they want to compete to show who can do the most for the client. Unfortunately, it is the client who usually loses in this situation.

What can we do to overcome these problems or to prevent them from arising in the first place? The NARC monograph suggests that conflicts between families and professionals or between different groups of professionals need to be directly confronted. More specifically, Shaffer and Bell (1978) suggest that the roles of everyone involved with planning for an individual must be clarified so that everyone knows who is supposed to do what with respect to setting goals and implementing ways of achieving them. They also suggest avoiding the use of jargon or vague overgeneralized statements during such meetings and particularly emphasize that everyone involved in the programming process needs to be heard. Attention must be paid to nonverbal communication as well as to what people are saying. It is also important to schedule meetings at appropriate times and locations for all involved participants and to provide encouragement for everyone involved to participate in planning meetings.

INFORMATION RESOURCES

Organizations and Journals

It has been said that there are two kinds of knowledge: the things that you know and carry around with you and the things that you know how to find out. This section is devoted to making the second kind of information accessible to you. It is extremely important in the provision of services to the handicapped to be able to find the kind of information that you don't know and don't carry around with you. There are two reasons for this. First, there is simply too much information available for any one person to master all of it. Therefore, it is important for everyone in the business of providing services to developmentally disabled people to know what they don't know and how to find it. The second reason is that more is learned daily about how to provide effective services. Hence, completion of a single training program, no matter how sophisticated and advanced, is not sufficient training in this field. Rather, it is necessary to stay current with respect to new findings and new techniques for providing good services.

One of the most common ways of keeping in touch with new developments in a field is to become a member of a professional organization in that field. There are four key functions that most professional organizations provide (there are, of course, a variety of additional functions provided by professional organizations that will not be discussed here). The first of these is publication of professional journals. Reading professional journals is one of the most important ways that professionals stay current with respect to the findings in their field. This is because professional journals publish new research findings as they become available. The second function that nearly all professional organizations provide is the organization and sponsorship of regular conventions, most often at the national level but frequently at regional and/or state levels as well. Conventions provide an opportunity to learn about new research findings, to discuss issues of concern with other people interested in the same topics, to find out what other people in the field are doing, and, of course, to get away from it all and have a good time. Most professional organizations also provide employment listings of jobs available, usually either in a publication such as a journal or at a convention, or both. Finally, membership in a professional organization makes you a member of a group of people who share the same pressures and concerns.

Naturally, it is unrealistic to expect anyone engaged in the business of providing direct services to belong to every relevant professional organization or keep up on all of the potentially useful literature. The annotated listing of organizations and journals that follows is intended to give you a selection from which to choose. We suggest that you obtain materials from these organizations describing their activities and services. Also, take a look at an issue or two of the journals that might interest you, and choose those organizations and/or journals that you feel are worth an investment of your time and money.

Exceptionality Organizations

These organizations are all concerned with various types of exceptional individuals.

The American Association on Mental
   Deficiency (AAMD)
5101 Wisconsin Avenue, N.W.
Washington, D.C. 20016

> AAMD is an interdisciplinary organization concerned with mental retardation. It publishes two journals, *Mental Retardation* and the *American Journal of Mental*

Deficiency. *Mental Retardation* is the more applied journal and therefore more likely to be of use to people directly providing services. AAMD also sponsors a yearly national convention, as well as conventions at the regional and state level. It has special interest groups, called divisions, in the areas of administration, education, psychology, private residential facilities, speech pathology and audiology, medicine, nursing, religion, resident living, social work, and vocational rehabilitation, as well as a general division.

The Association for the Severely
  Handicapped (TASH)
7010 Roosevelt Way, N.E.
Seattle, Washington 98115

This relatively new organization is also an interdisciplinary organization, and is composed of individuals who are concerned with the provision of quality services to the severely and profoundly handicapped. TASH publishes both a monthly newsletter that includes job availability notices and a quarterly journal *JASH* *(Journal of the Association for the Severely Handicapped)*. TASH also sponsors publication of various volumes that address issues of concern for the severely handicapped population. An annual conference is held every fall.

The Council for Exceptional Children
  (CEC)
1920 Association Drive
Reston, Virginia 22091

CEC is an organization composed of individuals who are concerned with the provision of special education services to a variety of exceptional populations. CEC sponsors a national convention and publishes the journals *Exceptional Children* and *Teaching Exceptional Children*. In addition, CEC has the following divisions: the Council of Administrators of Special Education; the Council for Children with Behavioral Disorders; the Division on Mental Retardation, which publishes the quarterly journal *Education and Training of the Mentally Retarded;* the Division for Children with Learning Disabilities; the Council for Educational Diagnostic Services; the Division for Early Childhood; the Division for Children with Communication Disorders; the Division on the Physically Handicapped, Homebound and Hospitalized; the Division for the Visually Handicapped; the Association for the Gifted; and the Teacher Education Division.

The organizations described above are probably the most influential professional organizations specifically concerned with developmental disabilities. The following seven organizations, all of which tend to be more consumer oriented and run, also share similar concerns.

The National Association for Retarded
  Citizens (NARC)
2709 Avenue E East
P.O. Box 6109
Arlington, Texas 76011

The National Society for Autistic
  Children
1234 Massachusetts Avenue, N.W.
Suite 107
Washington, D.C. 20005

The United Cerebral Palsy Association
66 East 34th Street, Third Floor
New York, New York 10016

The Epilepsy Foundation of America
1828 L Street, N.W., Suite 406
Washington, D.C. 20036

The American Coalition for Citizens
with Disabilities
1200 15th Street, N.W., Suite 201
Washington, D.C. 20005

The National Easter Seal Society for
Crippled Children and Adults
2023 West Ogden Avenue
Chicago, Illinois 60612

The March of Dimes Birth Defects
Foundation
1275 Mamoroneck Avenue
White Plains, New York 10605

Behavior Management Organizations

The Association for Behavior Analysis
(ABA)
Psychology Department
Western Michigan University
Kalamazoo, Michigan 49008

> ABA is an interdisciplinary organization that is concerned with theoretical, experimental, and applied analyses of behavior. A great many individuals associated with the field of applied behavior analysis are working to develop new procedures for serving developmentally disabled persons. ABA publishes a journal, *the Behavior Analyst,* that is devoted to discussions of issues in the field, and sponsors an annual convention every year during late spring or early summer.

The Association for the Advancement
of Behavior Therapy (AABT)
420 Lexington Avenue
New York, New York 10017

> AABT describes itself as a group for the clinical application of the principles of behavior modification. It publishes two quarterly journals, *Behavior Therapy* and *Behavioral Assessment,* and sponsors a yearly convention usually held in November or December.

A Rehabilitation Association

The National Rehabilitation Association
(NRA)
1522 K Street, N.W.
Washington, D.C. 20005

> The purpose of the NRA is to advance the rehabilitation of all handicapped persons. Included in its activities are a yearly convention and the publication of the *Journal of Rehabilitation.* The NRA has the following divisions: the Job Placement Division, which publishes the *Job Placement Digest;* the National Association for Independent Living; the National Association of Rehabilitation Instructors; the National Association of Rehabilitation Secretaries; the National Rehabilitation Administration Association, which publishes the *Journal of Rehabilitation Administration;* the National Rehabilitation Counseling Association, which publishes a newsletter and the *Journal of Applied Rehabilitation Counseling,* and the Vocational Evaluation and Work Adjustment Association, which publishes both a newsletter and a journal, the *VEWAA Bulletin.*

Other Professional Journals

In addition to the journals published by professional organizations, there is also a wide variety of other journals available published under the auspices of various commercial publishers or universities. It would be impossible to list all such available journals. However, some that you might find useful are:

Behavior Modification
Sage Publications, Inc.
275 South Beverly Drive
Beverly Hills, California 90212

The Journal of Applied Behavior
  Analysis
Mary Louise Wright, Business Officer
Department of Human Development
University of Kansas
Lawrence, Kansas 66045

Education and Treatment of Children
Presley Ridge School
530 Marshall Avenue
Pittsburgh, Pennsylvania 15214

OTHER INFORMATION SOURCES

There are a variety of other information sources besides professional organizations. Any good college or university library will have a collection that includes at least some of the journals in which you may be interested. It will also have access to the collections of other university libraries through an interlibrary loan service and may have access to computerized data bases such as ERIC abstracts and Psychological Abstracts.

There are two kinds of programs connected with universities in which you are likely to find the most extensive collections of materials related to programming for the developmentally disabled. The first type of program is called a Research and Training Center. There are a large number of these centers across the country. Three that specialize in mental retardation are located at the University of Wisconsin–Madison, the University of Oregon–Eugene, and Texas Technical University in Lubbock. The other type of special program to look for is called a University Affiliated Program (UAP). There are over 40 UAPs associated with universities across the United States. Each of these facilities is devoted to training, service, and research in relation to developmentally disabled persons.

There are many other information centers around the country that provide useful materials. Some that may be useful to you are:

The Center for Innovation and Teaching
  the Handicapped
Indiana University
2805 East 10th Street
Bloomington, Indiana 47401

The Handicapped Learner Materials
  Distribution Center
Indiana University
Bloomington, Indiana 47405

The National Clearinghouse of
Rehabilitation Training Materials
Oklahoma State University
115 Old USDA Building
Stillwater, Oklahoma 74074

The National Information Center for
Special Education Media
University of Southern California
University Park
3716 South Hope Street
Los Angeles, California 90007

The National Media Materials Center
for Severely Handicapped Persons
Peabody College
Box 318
Nashville, Tennessee 37203

The National Rehabilitation
Information Center
308 Muland Library
The Catholic University of America
Washington, D.C. 20064

Training Materials Information
Collection at ISMRDD
State and Community Services Division
University of Michigan
130 South First Street
Ann Arbor, Michigan 48104

SUGGESTED ACTIVITIES

1. What are the types of professional services that your agency uses regularly?
2. What community resources are you now using as aids to programming for your clients? How might you improve the use of these resources, possibly by improving communication?
3. What client needs have you identified in the last few months that your agency is not capable of meeting? What community resources do you have available that might help you to meet those needs? Develop a plan for making contact with those resources and developing a cooperative relationship with them that will benefit your clients.
4. Write to any of the organizations described in this chapter. Ask what they can do for you. Join as many organizations as you (a) feel will be helpful, and (b) can afford to join.
5. Go to the nearest university library and look at recent issues of the journals described in this chapter. Identify those journals that can be useful to you. Arrange to read them regularly by either going to the library every month or two or by subscribing to them.
6. Pick out a work-related topic for which you need more information. Call or write to several of the information sources described in this chapter and ask them what information they can give on that topic.

ADDITIONAL RESOURCES

Flynn, R. J., & Nitsch, K. E. (Eds.). *Normalization, social integration, and community services*. Baltimore: University Park Press, 1980.
Magrab, P. R., & Elder, J. O. (Eds.). *Planning for services to handicapped persons: Community, education, health*. Baltimore: Paul H. Brookes Publishing Co., 1979.
Riddell, R. Life with my retarded son: The hardest part is how the world treats us... *MS.*, 1980, *9*, 84, 86, 89.

REFERENCES

Elder, J. O. Essential components in development of interagency collaboration. In J. O. Elder & P. R. Magrab (Eds.), *Coordinating services to handicapped children.* Baltimore: Paul H. Brookes Publishers, 1980.

Gottlieb, J. Public, peer, and professional attitudes toward mentally retarded persons. In M. J. Begab & S. A. Richardson (Eds.), *The mentally retarded and society: A social science perspective.* Baltimore: University Park Press, 1975.

Hall, H. B. The intangible human factor: The most critical coordination variable. In J. O. Elder & P. R. Magrab (Eds.), *Coordinating services to handicapped children.* Baltimore: Paul H. Brookes Publishers, 1980.

Laten, S. M., & Wikler, L. *Behavioral social work assessment and intervention with families of the retarded.* Presented at the meeting of the Midwestern Association for Behavior Analysis, Chicago, 1978.

National Association for Retarded Citizens. *Citizen advocacy for mentally retarded children: An introduction.* Washington, D.C.: NARC, 1974.

National Association for Retarded Citizens. *The parent/professional partnership. The partnership: How to make it work.* Arlington, Tex.: NARC, 1977.

Shaffer, J. D., & Bell, J. E. *Parents and educators: Partners in individualized education program planning for handicapped students.* Des Moines: Midwest Regional Resource Center, 1978.

Index

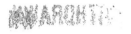